He wants sex.
She wants romance.

Sometimes it seems as if our partners are from different planets, as if he's from Mars and she's from Venus. In the bedroom, it is obvious that men and women are different, but we may not realize just how different we are. It is only through understanding and accepting our obvious and less obvious differences that we can achieve true intimacy and great sex . . .

·While many useful books address the mechanics of sex, this book addresses the mechanics of making sure you have sex. Through new approaches for communicating you will learn how to initiate sex in ways that assure that both your sexual needs and your partner's are satisfied. In addition, we will explore the psychological differences between men and women in a way that will help you understand what works best for your partner.

Most books focus on what men and women physically need, but few address their unique psychological needs as well. This book leads men and women toward sexual fulfillment both physically and emotionally.

John Gray

Other Books by John Gray, Ph.D.

What You Feel, You Can Heal:
A Guide for Enriching Relationships

Men, Women and Relationships:
Making Peace with the Opposite Sex

Men Are from Mars, Women Are from Venus:
A Practical Guide for Improving Communication
and Getting What You Want in Your Relationships

What Your Mother Couldn't Tell You & Your
Father Didn't Know: Advanced Relationship Skills
for Better Communication and Lasting Intimacy

Mars and Venus Together Forever:
Relationship Skills for Lasting Love

Mars and Venus in Love: Inspiring and
Heartfelt Stories of Relationships that Work

Mars AND Venus

IN THE Bedroom

A Guide to Lasting Romance and Passion

JOHN GRAY, Ph.D.

HarperTorch
An Imprint of HarperCollinsPublishers

HARPERTORCH
An Imprint of HarperCollins*Publishers*
10 East 53rd Street
New York, New York 10022-5299

Copyright © 1995, 2001 by J.G. Productions, Inc.
ISBN: 0-06-101571-7

First HarperTorch mass market paperback printing: September 2001
First HarperCollins trade paperback printing: February 1996
First HarperCollins hardcover printing: April 1995

HarperCollins ®, HarperTorch™, and ❦™ are trademarks of Harper-Collins Publishers Inc.

Printed in the United States of America

Visit HarperTorch on the World Wide Web at www.harpercollins.com

10

This book is dedicated to my wife, Bonnie,
whose openness, creativity, and love
continue to inspire my writings
and deepen my understanding of relationships.

Contents

Acknowledgments

I thank my wife, Bonnie, for once again sharing the journey of developing a book with me. I thank her for her continued patience and creative support in helping me to be successful as a loving partner. I also thank her for allowing me to share our stories and especially for continuing to expand my understanding and ability to honor the female perspective. Her insightful suggestions and comments have provided an important and necessary balance.

I thank my agent, Patti Breitman, for her helpful assistance, brilliant creativity, and enthusiasm, which have guided this book from its conception to its completion. She is a special angel in my life. I thank Carole Bidnick who connected Patti and me for the beginning of our first project, *Men Are from Mars, Women Are from Venus*.

I thank Nancy Peske for her persistent editorial expertise and creativity throughout the whole process. I thank Jack McKeown for his interest and committed support of this project since its beginning and for the support of the entire staff at HarperCollins for their continued responsiveness to my needs.

I thank Michael Najarian and his wife, Susan, for the successful organization of so many seminars. I thank Michael for the many extra hours of creative planning, plus the important and insightful feedback he has given me in developing this material. I thank the many different promoters and organizers who have put their hearts and souls into producing and supporting seminars for me to teach and develop the material in this book: Elly and Ian Coren in Santa Cruz; Ellis and Consuelo Goldfrit in Santa Cruz; Sandee Mac in Houston; Richi and Debra Mudd in Honolulu; Garry Francell of Heart

Acknowledgments

Seminars in Honolulu; Bill and Judy Elbring of *Life Partners* in San Francisco; David Farlow and Julie Ricksacker in San Diego; David and Marci Obstfeld in Detroit; Fred Kleiner and Mary Wright in Washington, D.C.; Clark and Dotti Bartells in Seattle; Earlene and Jim Carillo in Las Vegas; Bart and Merril Berens in L.A.; and Grace Merrick of the Dallas Unity Church.

I thank John Vestman at Trianon Studios for his expert audio recordings of my seminars. I thank Dave Morton and the staff of Cassette Express for their continued appreciation of this material and their quality service. I thank Bonnie Solow for her competence and gentle support in producing the audio version of this book, as well as the staff at HarperAudio.

I thank Ramy El-Batrawi of Genesis-Nuborn Productions and his wife, Ronda, for the successful creation and ongoing production of television infomercials making available audio and video presentations of my seminars.

〜

I thank my executive assistants, Ariana Husband and Susie Harris, for their hard work, devotion, and efficient managing of my schedule and office.

I thank my chiropractor, Terry Safford, for the incredible support he provided twice a week during the most intensive six months of this project. I thank Raymond Himmel for his many acupuncture sessions at the end of this project that miraculously healed me of dizziness and exhaustion. I thank my friend Renee Swisko for her amazing and powerful healing sessions with me and the rest of my family.

I thank my friends and associates for their open, honest, and supportive sharing of ideas and feedback: Clifford McGuire, Jim Kennedy and Anna Everest, John and Bonnie Grey, Reggie and Andrea Henkart, Lee and Joyce Shapiro, Gabriel Grunfeld, Harold Bloomfield and Sirah Vittese, Jordan Paul, Lenny Eiger, Charles Wood, Jacques Earley, Chris Johns, Mike Bosch and Doug Aarons.

I thank Oprah for her warm and personal support and the opportunity to share freely

Acknowledgments

〜

my ideas on her show before 30 million viewers.

I thank the thousands of participants of my relationship seminars who shared their stories and encouraged me to write this book. Their positive and loving support along with the thousands of calls and letters I have received from readers continues to support me in developing and validating the principles of this book.

Particularly for the enormous success of my previous books I wish to thank the millions of readers who not only have shared my books with others but continue to benefit from these ideas in their lives and relationships.

I give thanks to God for the opportunity to make a difference in this world and the simple but effective wisdom that comes to me and is presented in this book.

Introduction

He wants sex. She wants romance. Sometimes it seems as if our partners are from different planets, as if he's from Mars and she's from Venus. In the bedroom, it is obvious that men and women are different, but we may not realize just how different we are. It is only through understanding and accepting our obvious and less obvious differences that we can achieve true intimacy and great sex.

Why Sex Is So Important

We're all aware that sex tends to be more important to men while romance is more important to women, but we generally don't understand why. Without a deeper understanding of this fundamental difference, women commonly underestimate the importance of sex for men and many times judge them as superficial for wanting only one thing.

A woman's judgments begin to soften when she discovers the real reasons that some men seem to want only sex. With a deeper understanding of our sexual differences based on our historical development and social conditioning, she can begin to understand why, for many men, sexual arousal is the key for helping them connect with and realize their loving feelings.

❧

For many men, sexual arousal is the key for helping them connect with and realize their loving feelings.

❧

It is through sex that a man's heart opens, allowing him to experience both his loving

参

feelings and his hunger for love as well. Ironically, it is sex that allows a man to feel his needs for love, while it is receiving love that helps a woman to feel her hunger for sex.

⤸

Sex allows a man to feel his needs for love, while receiving love helps a woman to feel her hunger for sex.

⤸

A man often misunderstands a woman's real need for romance and may feel instead that she is withholding sex. When he wants sex and she is not readily in the mood, he easily misunderstands and feels rejected. He does not instinctively realize that a woman generally needs to feel loved and romanced before she can feel her hunger for sex.

Just as a woman needs good communication with her partner to feel loved and loving, a man needs sex. Certainly, a man can feel loved in other ways, but the most powerful way a woman's love can touch his soul and open his heart is through great sex.

〜 What Makes Sex Great

Ideally, for sex to be great there must be loving and supportive communication in the relationship. This is the first step. When communication works, all the bedroom skills in this book can be most easily applied.

If communication in a relationship is OK, hearing and using the ideas in this book will dramatically increase the passion and quality of sex. When sex gets better, suddenly the whole relationship gets better. Through great sex, the man begins to feel more love, and, as a result, the woman starts getting the love she may have been missing. Automatically, communication and intimacy increase.

Introduction

∽

∽

When sex gets better, suddenly the whole relationship automatically gets better.

∽

When a couple is experiencing relationship problems, sometimes, instead of focusing on the problems, taking a shortcut and creating great sex immediately reduces the problems and makes them easier to solve. To most effectively solve relationship problems and ensure lasting intimacy and better communication, I recommend that you read my other books, *Men Are from Mars, Women Are from Venus* and *Mars and Venus Together Forever*. Sometimes, however, the most effective way to jumpstart a relationship is to first learn the bedroom skills for creating great sex.

Great sex is the most powerful way to open a man's heart and help him to feel his love and express it to a woman. Great sex softens a woman's heart and helps her to relax and receive her partner's support in other areas of the relationship. This softening of her feelings dramatically improves her ability to communicate in a manner that her partner can hear without becoming defensive. This improved communication in turn provides a basis for sex to remain passionate.

&

Great sex is the most powerful way to open a man's heart and help him to feel his love and express it to a woman.

&

& Why Another Book on Sex?

While many useful books address the mechanics of sex, this book addresses the mechanics of making sure you have sex. Through new approaches for communicating, you will learn how to initiate sex in ways that assure that both your sexual needs and your partner's are satisfied. In addition, we will explore the psychological differences between men and women in a way that will help you understand what works best for your partner.

Most books focus on what men and women physically need, but few address their unique psychological needs as well. This book leads men and women toward sexual fulfillment both physically and emotionally. Not only are men grateful when women learn this information, but women experience greater happiness in and out of the bedroom. I receive so many letters from couples after they take my seminars saying that they are now enjoying the best sex they ever had. Sometimes these couples have been married only a few years, but some of them have been married for more than thirty years.

〜 Advanced Bedroom Skills

Women today expect more from sex than ever before. It used to be that sex was primarily a way a woman fulfilled her husband. For many of our mothers, sex was something she did for him and not for herself. But now that birth control is more reliable and available and society is much more accepting of women's sexual needs and desires, women have greater permission to explore and enjoy their sensual side. For many women, a growing interest in sex also reflects their need to find balance within themselves by reconnecting with their feminine side.

Having spent most of the day in a traditionally male job, she too wants a "wife" to greet *her* with love when she gets home. She too wants to enjoy the release that sex brings. Great sex fulfills her as much as it fulfills him. To cope with the stress of the modern workplace, not only does he need her support, but she needs his as well. Through learning new relationship skills,

men and women can solve this problem together.

Advanced bedroom skills are required if a
man is to provide his partner with the sexual
fulfillment that she now requires. The more
traditional bedroom skills men and women
have used for centuries are outdated. It is
not enough for a man to have his way with a
woman. She wants more. She wants pleasure too. He must learn her way as well.

Just as women want more, men also want
more. Men don't want to give up passion in
their relationships. More and more, both
men and women would rather get a divorce
than stay in a passionless marriage.

Neither sex is willing to put up with the
old system of a man having discreet affairs
to fulfill his sexual passion while a woman
sacrifices her need for passion in favor of
maintaining the family unit. AIDS and other
sexually transmitted diseases make extra-
marital affairs far more dangerous than they
were in the past. A modern man wants his
partner to value sex in a way that allows him

to stay passionately connected to her and their relationship. To achieve this end, advanced bedroom skills are required for both men and women.

In the first twelve chapters of *Mars and Venus in the Bedroom*, we will explore how to create great sex in bed, and then, in chapter 13, we will explore the importance of romance outside the bedroom to keep the passion alive.

᙭ Why Couples Stop Having Sex

Quite commonly, after being married for several years, one of the partners stops wanting sex. Although the partner feels as if he or she has simply lost interest in sex, the disinterest is really caused because certain conditions for wanting sex are not being met. Throughout *Mars and Venus in the Bedroom*, we will explore these different needs in much detail. Many times men and women do not clearly know what their needs are or how to have them met. Rather than feel frustrated all the time, they just lose interest.

Surprisingly, at my seminars it is mostly the women who come up to me during the breaks and mention that their husbands just aren't interested in sex anymore. Certainly, it is not unusual for men to want sex more than their partners do, but no matter which partner loses interest, passion can be rekindled with advanced bedroom skills.

∽ How to Share This Book with Your Partner

This is a fun book and not too technical. I purposely made many of the chapters very short so that you can put the book down and enjoy practicing some of these new bedroom skills.

If a woman suggests to a man that he read this book, it is important that she not give him the message that he needs it or that she wants to improve their sex life. It may sound too serious to him and convey the message that *he* is not good enough or that *he* needs to be improved; he'll easily feel insulted by this approach.

Instead, she should say, "Let's read this book about sex. It is really fun," or "This is really a sexy book. Let's take turns reading it together." He'll respond much more positively if he sees that she wants to try something new along with him.

When a man approaches a woman to read this book, he should use the same approach but also be careful not to insist. If she resists, he can read it on his own and begin to use many of the techniques involved. As he succeeds in applying these techniques, she will be much more willing to read the book.

In each case, if your partner resists, gracefully say OK and read the book yourself. Eventually, the man will become interested in what the woman is reading if he sees that she is working on making sex great. Likewise, the woman will be more interested in sharing the book when the man begins applying new skills.

If your partner does not seem interested, just leave the book around the bedroom or put it in the bathroom, and curiosity will motivate him or her without you having to do anything more.

Reading this book out loud with your partner can assist you in expressing feelings about sex in an easy manner. By making a simple sound of enthusiasm or delight as a certain passage is read, you can give your partner a very important message. In a positive way, you can share ideas that you have avoided expressing for fear that they might sound critical or controlling. Seeing something in print makes it much easier to accept.

Another approach is for both partners to read the book alone and then start using it. Eventually, it is helpful to improve communication if they read it out loud together or at least read their favorite parts.

Many times a woman is hesitant to describe what she likes in sex because she doesn't want her partner to follow her instructions mechanically. Reading about various skills in sex will certainly give both men and women plenty of new approaches to experiment with. This newness can assist couples in experiencing new passion. The purpose of this book is not just to educate, but also to inspire.

Men sometimes tell me that they already know what I am telling them about sex, but it is certainly great to be reminded in such a positive way. Just talking about sex or reading about it in a book can release new passion.

I recommend that, after trying out some of these approaches, a couple continue to talk occasionally about each of their unique preferences. Some of these skills or approaches may be desirable to you but not to your partner. In some cases, over time your partner may change and begin to like certain things and not like other things.

It is important that you do not demand something that makes your partner uncomfortable and do not do something to your partner that he or she doesn't want. Sex is a precious gift that two people can give to each other when they love each other.

It is best to just take in this information and then use whatever you like, as if choosing from a buffet. What some people like, others don't like. You would never want to convince your partner that she should like potatoes if she doesn't, nor would you judge your partner if he likes potatoes and you don't.

For sex and passion to grow over time, it is important that we not feel the possibility of being judged or criticized for our wishes and desires. We should always try to approach sex in a nonjudgmental manner.

I offer this book as a reminder of many of the things you probably already know intuitively. I personally have benefited tremendously from each of the ideas I present, as have thousands of people I've counseled or who have attended my seminars. I hope you enjoy this book and continue to enjoy its insights for the rest of your days and nights.

Great sex is God's gift to those who are

committed to creating loving and supportive relationships. Great sex is your reward, and you deserve it.

> John Gray
> April 29, 1994

Special Note

This book is for couples who are in a committed, monogamous relationship. If you are not in a committed, monogamous relationship, or if you are not absolutely one-hundred-percent sure that your partner is HIV negative, for your own safety and self-respect, you must practice safe sex. Many books explain how to practice safe sex without sacrificing spontaneity and pleasure, and I urge you to learn how to protect yourself from the AIDS virus as well as other sexually transmitted diseases.

It is especially important for women to take precautions. In a heterosexual relationship, women are at a higher risk than men are to be exposed to the AIDS virus, because the virus can enter her bloodstream through tiny tears in her vagina, tears that commonly occur during intercourse. Some women find it very difficult to insist that a man use a condom every time they have sex to protect her. Women need to remember that their lives and their health are far too important to risk just because he doesn't want to reduce his sensitivity by wearing a condom. Many brands of condoms and lubricants will limit the loss of sensitivity, and there are many enjoyable ways of incorporating condoms into sex. Also, when a man's sensitivity is reduced by wearing a condom, he may have an easier time holding back from climaxing too early before she is satisfied, and by holding back, as I explain in greater detail in chapter 9, his orgasm may be even stronger.

Men need to remember that it is extremely difficult for a woman to relax, trust her partner, and truly enjoy sex when she is worried about being infected by HIV or another sexually transmitted disease, or when she is worried about getting pregnant. In the heat of the moment, it is easy for a man to forget the consequences of unsafe sex, but if he takes responsibility for remembering to protect her *every* time, she will appreciate him greatly and be even more open and intimate during sex because she will feel safe.

If you are in a committed, monogamous partnership and have been for at least six months, you can be accurately tested for the HIV virus (it often does not show up in the blood until six months after exposure). Ask your doctor or a public health clinic to test you and your partner.

CHAPTER 1

Advanced Bedroom Skills for Great Sex

One of the special rewards for learning and applying advanced bedroom skills is that sex gets better and better. Like a fabulous vacation after working hard, or a sensual walk through the forest on a sunny spring day, or the exhilaration of climbing to the top of a mountain, great sex is not just a reward but something that can rejuvenate the body, mind, and soul. It brightens our days and strengthens our relationship in the most basic ways.

A great sex life is not just the symptom of a passionate relationship, but is also a major factor in creating it. Great sex fills our hearts with love and can fulfill almost all our emotional needs. Loving sex, passionate sex, sensual sex, long sex, short sex, quick sex, gourmet sex, playful sex, tender sex, soft sex, hard sex, romantic sex, goal-oriented sex, erotic sex, simple sex, cool sex, and hot sex are all an important part of keeping the passion of love alive.

↝

A *great sex life* is not just the symptom of a passionate relationship, but is also a major factor in creating it.

↝

↝ Great Sex for Women

Great sex softens a woman and opens her to experience the love in her heart and to re-member her partner's love for her in a most definite way. Her partner's skillful and knowing touch leaves no doubt in her mind that she is important to him. The hunger for love within her soul is fulfilled with her partner's passionate and fully present attention. An ever-present tension is momentarily released as she surrenders once again to the deepest longings of her feminine being. Her passion to love and be loved can be fully felt and fulfilled.

◡ Great Sex for Men

Great sex releases a man from all his frustrations and allows him to rekindle his passion and commitment to the relationship. In a most immediate way, he experiences the results of his efforts. Her fulfillment is his ultimate quest and victory. Her warm responsiveness excites, electrifies, and awakens the deepest fibers of his masculine being. Heaven's gates are opened, and he has arrived! Through her fulfillment, he feels he has made his mark and his love is appreciated. His sometimes hidden but all-consuming and ever-present desire to love and be loved is both felt and satisfied as he returns to his world yet remains deep within her.

∽ **Great Sex for the Relationship**

Great sex reminds both men and women of the tender and highest love that originally drew them together. The alchemy of great sex generates the chemicals in the brain and body that allow the fullest enjoyment of one's partner. It increases our attraction to each other, stimulates greater energy, and even promotes better health.* It leaves us not only with the sparkle of youthful vitality, but with a heightened sense of beauty, wonder, and appreciation not only for each other, but for the world around us. Great sex is God's special gift to those who

*In his book, *The Power of Five*, Harold Bloomfield, M.D., reveals that regular sex is vital for maintaining higher estrogen levels in women. Higher estrogen has been associated with better bones, better cardiovascular health, and a feeling of joy in life. Men who experience regular sex have a higher testosterone level, which leads to greater confidence, vitality, strength, and energy.

work hard to make love a priority in their lives.

The one major characteristic that makes a marriage more than just a loving friendship is sex. Sex directly nurtures our male and female sides more than any other activity a couple can share. Great sex is soothing to a woman and helps keep her in touch with her feminine side, while it strengthens a man and keeps him in touch with his masculine side. Sex has a tremendous power to bring us closer or push us apart.

To create great sex, it is not enough for men or women to follow their ancient instincts. As times have changed, the quality of sex has become much more important. Our mothers couldn't tell us and our fathers didn't know the secrets of great sex. Just as the skills for relating and communicating have changed, so also have the skills for sex. To fulfill our partners in bed, new skills are required.

Without a clear understanding of our different requirements in sex, after a few years—sometimes only months—sex becomes routine and mechanical. By making a few but significant shifts, we can completely overcome this pattern.

〜 **Women Love Great Sex**

Great sex requires a positive attitude about sex. For a man to continue feeling attracted to his partner, he needs to feel that she likes sex as much as he does. Quite often a man will feel defeated in sex because he mistakenly gets the message that his partner is not as interested in it. Without a deeper understanding of how we are wired differently for sex, it is very easy to feel discouraged.

Women love great sex as much as men. The difference between a woman and a man is that she doesn't feel her strong desire for sex unless her need for love is first satisfied. Most important, she first needs to feel loved and special to a man. When her heart is opened in this way, her sexual center begins to open, and she feels a longing equal to or greater than what any man feels. To her, love is much more important than sex, but as the need for love is fulfilled, the importance of sex dramatically increases.

〜

Women love great sex as much as men, but to feel turned on, women have many more requirements.

〜

Even if a woman doesn't feel loved but feels the possibility of being loved, she can begin to feel her deep desires for sex. Generally speaking, however, a man needs only the opportunity and the place to become aroused. In the beginning of a relationship, sexual arousal is much more automatic and quick for a man.

∽

**In the beginning of a relationship,
sexual arousal is much more automatic
and quick for a man.**

∽

∽ **Different Chemistry**

This difference is reflected physiologically.
The hormones in a man's body that are responsible for arousal quickly build up and
then are quickly released after orgasm. For a
woman, the pleasure builds up much more
slowly and remains long after orgasm.

For a woman, arousal slowly builds long
before it becomes a physical desire for sex.
Before longing for sexual stimulation, a
woman first feels warm, sensual, and attractive. She feels drawn to a man and enjoys
sharing time together. It could be days before she wants to have sex.

⤳

**For a woman, arousal slowly builds long
before it becomes a physical desire for
sex. It is hard for a man to understand
her different requirements because they
are not his experience.**

⤳

When a man becomes aroused, it is immediately sexual. To wait days requires enormous restraint on his part. It is hard for him to understand her different requirements because they are not his experience.

When a man returns home from a trip, he might want to have sex immediately, while his wife wants to take some time to get reacquainted and talk. Without an understanding of this difference, it would be very easy for him to feel unnecessarily rejected or for her to feel used.

In the beginning of a relationship, a man is more understanding of a woman's need to wait before she has sex. But once they are having sex, he doesn't realize that she still requires emotional support first before she wants to have sex. In a very real sense, emotional support is the price of admission. He does not understand the importance of fulfilling her emotional needs first because his requirements are less.

〰 **"Men Only Want One Thing"**

Women commonly think men only want one thing: sex. The truth is, however, that men really want love. A man wants love just as much as a woman, but before he can open his heart and let in his partner's love, sexual arousal is a prerequisite. Just as a woman needs love to open up to sex, a man needs sex to open up to love.

෴

Just as a woman needs love to open up to sex, a man needs sex to open up to love.

෴

As a general guideline, a woman needs to be emotionally fulfilled *before* she can long for sexual contact. A man, however, gets much of his emotional fulfillment *during* sex.

Women do not understand this about men. The hidden reason a man is so much in a hurry to have sex is that through sex, a man is able to feel again. Throughout the day, a man becomes so focused on his work that he loses touch with his loving feelings. Sex helps him to feel again. Through sex, a man's heart begins to open up. Through sex, a man can give and receive love the most.

When a woman begins to understand this difference, it changes her whole perspective on sex. Instead of a man's desire for sex being something crude and divorced from love, she can begin to see it as his way of eventually finding love. A woman's feelings about a man's preoccupation with sex can dramatically shift when she understands why a man needs sex.

∽ Why Men Need Sex

Men need sex to feel. For thousands of years, men adapted to their primary job as protector and provider by shutting down their sensitivities, emotions, and feelings. Getting the job done was more important than taking the time to explore feelings. More feeling or sensitivity would just hold them back or get in the way.

∽

Men need sex to feel.

∽

To go out into the wild or into battle, men needed to put their feelings aside. To provide for and protect their families, men were required to risk their lives while enduring the discomforts of scorching sun and freezing cold. Men gradually adapted to this requirement by becoming desensitized. In fact, this difference shows up dramatically in skin sensitivity. Women's skin is ten times more sensitive than men's skin.

To cope with pain, men learned to turn off their feelings. When they stopped feeling pain, however, they also lost their ability to feel pleasure and love. For many men, other than hitting their finger with a hammer or watching a football game, sex is one of the only ways they can feel! It is definitely the way they can feel most intensely. When a man is aroused, he rediscovers the love hidden in his heart. Through sex, a man can feel, and through feeling, he can come back to his soul again.

∽ Why Women Don't Understand

Women don't understand this difference because they have different requirements to fully feel. A woman primarily needs the emotional security to talk about her feelings. When she feels supported in a relationship, she can rediscover the love in her heart. When her emotional needs are met in this way, her sexual needs become more important.

It is confusing to her when he wants sex and they are not even talking or he has ignored her for days. To her, it seems as if he doesn't care if they have much of a relationship. She has no idea that when he begins to hunger for sex it is because he wants to reconnect and share love. Just as communication is so important to women, sex is important to men.

A woman's sexual responsiveness is the most powerful way he can hear that he is loved. Sex can be the most powerful means to rekindle a man's feelings of love.

When Mom said that the way to a man's

heart was through his stomach, she was about four inches too high. Sex is the direct line to a man's heart.

❧

When Mom said that the way to a man's heart was through his stomach, she was about four inches too high.

❧

❧ **What Men Need**

A man is empowered and nurtured most when he feels appreciated, accepted, and trusted. When a woman is aroused, she is actually giving a man megadoses of what he needs most.

When a woman is longing to have sex with a man, she is most open and trusting. In a very dramatic way, she is willing to surrender her defenses and not only reveal her nakedness, but bring him into her body and being as well. By desiring a man in this way, she makes him feel very accepted. Then, when his every touch creates a pleasurable response, he feels greatly appreciated. In the most tangible and physical way possible, he feels and experiences that he is making a difference.

Even if he is stressed from the day, if his wife is feeling loved and supported and enjoys sex with him, he can be immediately rejuvenated. Although it seems as if sex makes him feel better, it is really that he is feeling again and able to let in her love. He is no longer cut off from his feeling self but can move into that deserted part of his being again. He can feel whole again. Like a thirsty man wandering in the desert, he can finally relax and take a drink from the oasis of his feelings.

∽

Like a thirsty man wandering in the desert, during sex he can finally relax and take a drink from the oasis of his feelings.

∽

Through touching her softness and entering the warmth of her loving body, he is able to remain hard and masculine but also experience his own softness and warmth. Through skillfully restraining his sexual passions, he is able to gradually open up not just to pleasurable sensations, but to the deeper joy of loving his partner and being loved in return.

∽ **What Makes Sex Great**

It was about the fifth year of my marriage with Bonnie when I began to understand consciously what really makes sex great.

One time after having really great sex, I said, "Wow, that was great. I loved it. I loved every little moment. That was as good as it was in the beginning . . ."

I looked at Bonnie, expecting her to nod in agreement or say something like, "Yes, that was spectacular." Instead, she looked a little puzzled.

I said, "Well, wasn't it as good for you?"

She said matter-of-factly, "I thought it was much better."

I suddenly had ambivalent feelings. I thought, "What do you mean, this was better? Were you just faking it in the beginning? How could you say this was better? Wasn't it great then too?"

She continued, "When we first had sex, it was wonderful, but you didn't really know me and I didn't really know you. It takes years to really get to know someone. Now when you make love to me, you know who I am. You know the best of me and you know the worst of me, and you still desire me and love me. That is what makes sex great for me now."

From that moment on, I began to realize the truth of what she said. What makes sex really great is love. The more you get to know someone and continue to grow in intimacy and love, the more the sexual experience has a chance to thrive.

Over the years, my sexual experience had also changed. It had been so gradual that I hadn't even noticed until she pointed it out. This awareness allowed me to focus my attention on how to make sex even better. In the next chapter, we will explore how sex can continue to improve.

CHAPTER 2

Sex and Passion

Without passion, sex becomes routine and boring. With the assistance of advanced bedroom skills and love, a couple can continue to experience great passion and fulfillment. Instead of becoming less passionate over the years, a man who sees and touches his wife's body can be more turned on than ever. Not only can he be excited by the pleasure of arousal and increasing sexual intensity, but he can also be aware of how much more love, warmth, passion, and sensual affection he will be able to experience as well as provide for her. This awareness elevates sex to an even higher level of passion and excitement.

When she feels his passion for her, she can

rejoice in his continued desire to connect with her and provide her with pleasure. She also recognizes sex as an opportunity to share love in a way that nurtures him the most. Sex becomes a beautiful expression of her love for him and an opportunity to receive in the deepest fibers of her femininity his love for her.

After practicing advanced bedroom skills, he will be much more aware that he is not only loving her, but also is getting the love he needs. He will be turned on to her not just because he is aroused, but because he loves her and wants to get close. Without depending on some fantasy woman to be turned on, he will truly know who he is loving.

Sex is great when it is shared in love and the love keeps growing. For a woman to grow in sexual fulfillment, she primarily needs to feel emotionally supported in the relationship, but it is also important for the man to skillfully understand her different sexual needs.

For a man to grow in sexual fulfillment, he

primarily needs to feel successful in fulfilling his partner sexually. This requires that he practice new skills not only in the relationship, but also in bed.

↬

For a woman to grow in sexual fulfillment, she primarily needs to feel emotionally supported in the relationship, but it is also important for the man to skillfully understand her different sexual needs.

↬

↬ **How Sex Can Get Better**

Sex can always get better, but like anything else, it requires new information and the opportunity to practice. Most men are never taught how to have sex. Once they can get turned on, they are somehow expected to be

sexual experts. Sure, they know the mechanics, but the art of giving a woman an orgasm is a different story altogether. How are
men supposed to know what makes women
happy when they are not women? For great
sex, a man needs to understand a woman's
body and what turns her on.

**How are men supposed to know
what makes women happy
when they are not women?**

It is hard for men to find out what makes
women really happy in bed because we are
expected to already know. In most cases, a
man actually thinks he does know. He mistakenly assumes that what makes him
happy will make her happy. When a woman
isn't satisfied, he thinks something is wrong
with her instead of with his techniques. He
doesn't understand that a woman's needs
are dramatically different from his in bed.

〜

〜

A man doesn't instinctively understand that a woman's sexual needs are dramatically different from his in bed. He mistakenly assumes that what makes him happy will make her happy.

〜

〜 Having Sex the First Time

I remember when I first had sex. My partner and I had talked about it and were going to go all the way. I was so excited. I immediately and instinctively began to run around the bases as quickly as possible to score.

I noticed that she was following another tactic. She didn't go right to my erogenous zone. It was as though she was purposely striking out. She was moving her hands slowly up and down my body. Down my thighs and then back up to my chest. Up and down my arms and then up and down my chest and back. She was touching me everywhere I didn't want to be touched. Since we were planning to go all the way, I reached down to her hand and put it between my legs. I said, "There!"

∽ Women Slow Up While Men Speed Up

I didn't understand at the time what she was doing. I thought she was trying to torture me. I didn't care about being touched all over my body. I just wanted to be touched in one place. Later on, as I learned about a woman's body, I discovered that she was doing to me what she would have liked me to do to her.

Men don't instinctively know what women like, and even when they hear about it, they tend to forget. Every song and book about sex says the same thing. A woman likes a man with a slow hand. Yet once he gets excited, he speeds up. He assumes she wants it speeded up because he does. He doesn't have a clue how much more exciting he can make it for her by restraining himself again and again.

෨

A woman likes a man with a slow hand.

෨

When he gets excited, he gives the kind of stimulation that he would like but not what she needs. To make sex great over time, a man needs to open his awareness to the different needs a woman has while a woman has to help her man be successful in fulfilling her sexually.

෨ How Sex Is Different for Men and Women

Sex is a very different experience for women and men. A man experiences pleasure primarily as a *release* of sexual tension. A woman experiences sex in an opposite way. For her, the great joys of sex correspond to a gradual *buildup* of tension. The more she can feel her desire for sex, the more fulfilling it is.

❧

A *man* experiences pleasure primarily as a release *of sexual tension*. A *woman's* pleasure corresponds to a gradual buildup *of sexual tension*.

❧

For a man, sex instinctively is a testosterone drive toward the ultimate release of climax. When he becomes aroused, he automatically seeks release. His fulfillment in sex is mainly associated with the release of tension leading to and including the orgasm.

Biologically, a man is always seeking release. Unlike a woman, whose sexual interest is generated through arousal, when a man is aroused, he is already seeking release. In a sense, he is trying to "empty out" while she is seeking to be "filled up."

A man's immediate desire to touch and be touched in his sensitive zones is a given. He does not need much help in getting excited. He needs help in releasing or letting go of his excitement. In a sense, he seeks to *end* his excitement, while a woman seeks to *extend* her excitement to feel more deeply her inner longing.

She relishes his ability to slowly build up her desire to be touched in her most sensitive zones. As one layer at a time is stripped away, she longs for the deeper layers of her sensual soul to be revealed. As much as he wants to immediately satisfy his desire for sexual stimulation, she hungers and loves to feel her desire increase.

〜 **Why Men Crave Release**

When the man touches the softness of a woman's bare breast, for example, he begins to feel his own inner link to experiencing pleasure and love. Through touching her soft femininity, he can connect with his own softness and yet remain masculine.

Sensuality is a part of his being, but he primarily experiences it through touching her body and feeling her pleasurable response. Many times after having great sex with my wife, I realize that I had forgotten how beautiful the trees are in our neighborhood. I go outside and breathe in the fresh air and feel alive again.

It is not that I didn't feel alive in my work, but by connecting with my wife through great sex, I can reawaken and bring to life my more sensual feelings that are easily forgotten in the focused pursuit of achieving my goals at work. In a sense, great sex helps me to stop and smell the flowers.

The more a man in his daily life is disconnected from his feelings, the more he will crave sexual stimulation and release. The intense pleasure of release at every stage of the sexual unfolding allows him to connect momentarily with his feelings and open his heart. For him, sexual hunger is not only for the experience of pleasure, but also for the experience of love.

Although he may not be aware of it, his persistent sexual longing is really his soul seeking wholeness. The barren landscape of living only in his mind seeks union with the rich, sensuous, colorful, and sweet-smelling terrain of his heart.

A man's persistent sexual longing is really his soul seeking wholeness. The barren landscape of living only in his mind seeks union with the rich, sensuous, colorful, and sweet-smelling terrain of his heart.

As his need to touch and be touched sexually is satisfied, his ability to *feel* automatically increases. As his feeling self is awakened, a tremendous energy is released. He can experience again his feelings of joy, love, and peace.

∽ **The Pleasure of Intercourse**

Before intercourse, a man longs to enter a woman's body. When he moves into her, his pleasure is greatly intensified. This pleasure results from the releasing of his sexual tension.

As he moves within her, his whole being is nourished. Suddenly, he is teleported out of the dry domain of his intellectual detachment into the moist caverns of sensitive and sensuous feeling.

∽

During intercourse, a man is teleported out of the dry domain of his intellectual detachment into the moist caverns of sensitive and sensuous feeling.

∽

A man's penis is his most sensitive organ; when it is touched, all of him is touched, soothed, excited, and electrified with pleasure. The feelings of love and attachment that are so easily dismissed by his rational mind are suddenly awakened by the intensity of sexual fulfillment.

After entering his partner, he feels the intense satisfaction of arriving at his goal. When his tension is released, he automatically experiences a wave of increased feeling.

After this momentary release of tension, he pulls back to experience the tension again and then plunges forward to release it. In this way, the tension builds up until he experiences a final release.

∽ How a Man Feels Love

A man is free to feel when he has achieved his goal. When his male side has done its work successfully, he swings over to his female side and fully feels. When he can satisfy his own desires and also fulfill his partner, he can relax and feel a greater sense of peace, love, and joy.

In a way, when he and his partner experience an orgasm, he feels he has completed his job and has been richly rewarded by her deeply felt appreciation and love for him.

By providing her orgasm first, a man opens a woman up to fully respond to his orgasm. After she has experienced her orgasm, she can best share the fullness of her love and receptivity. To whatever extent his partner loves him, at this precious moment, a man is able to let it in the most.

❧

To whatever extent his partner loves him, at the precious moment of orgasm, a man is able to receive her love the most.

❧

Particularly when he knows she is fulfilled and appreciative of him, he can fully thrive in that moment. More than at any other time, he can let her love in and can feel the love deep in his heart and reaffirm his commitment to her.

❧

As a man's heart opens during orgasm, he is able to feel the depth of his love and reaffirm his commitment to her.

❧

❧ The Therapy of Great Sex

Any resentments building up in a man are easily washed away when he experiences great sex. There is no therapy better for a man than great sex. Sometimes therapy or counseling is needed to get to that place where a man and woman can experience great sex, but once a couple is there and they know how to keep getting there, for a man great sex keeps him going and keeps the magic of passionate love alive.

Without the regular experience of great sex, it is very easy for a man to forget how much he loves his partner. He may wish her well and be congenial or civil in the relationship, but he will not feel the deep connection that they felt in the beginning.

Without great sex, her little imperfections will begin to get bigger and bigger in his eyes. Unlike a woman, who needs to talk about feelings to feel more loving, a man can feel more loving through great sex.

Although good communication is essential in a relationship and will lead to great sex, when a woman in a relationship doesn't experience great sex over time, she can easily harden under the weight of all her responsibilities. She feels responsible not only for herself, but also for her partner. She forgets her own sensual and sexual feminine desires. Without the romantic support of her loving companion, she doesn't feel she has time for herself.

～

～ Why Women Relish Desire

The more a woman is focused throughout her day on caring for and giving to others, the less aware she is of herself and her own sensual desires. She may be in touch with other people's feelings but out of touch with her own.

Just as a man forgets feelings, a woman forgets her sensual desires and longings. The practicalities of day-to-day survival and living take precedence over her deeper and more sensual desires. The more pressured or overwhelmed she is, the harder it is for her to relax and enjoy life's simple pleasures.

～

Just as a man forgets feelings, a woman forgets her sensual desires and longings. The practicalities of day-to-day survival and living take precedence over her deeper and more sensual desires.

～

When a man focuses on a woman in a caring and attentive way, he frees her to experience herself again. When a woman feels temporarily relieved of her pressure to care for others, she can begin to feel her sexual desires. A man's romantic attention to details designed to please her automatically begins to open her up.

By receiving the caring, nurturing, and sensuous support her female side craves, she begins to consciously feel her sexual yearnings. It is as though she doesn't even know she wants this stimulation until she gets it. The act of skillfully giving a woman what she needs helps her to discover her needs, and then she begins to long for more.

For example, when a man touches a woman close to her erogenous zones and then pulls away, back and forth in a rhythmic manner, a woman can begin to feel her desire to be touched more intensely. A skillful man moves his touch in the direction that she will eventually want him to touch, and then just as he gets close, he pulls away. This has the effect of increasing her desire for him to touch her there. He teases her by giving a little and then taking it away.

As a man touches her body in the nonerogenous zones bordering the places where she is not usually touched, she automatically begins to feel her need to be touched in the erogenous zones.

During great sex, a woman's desire gradually increases. In the beginning she may only feel a little or faint desire, but as that desire is fulfilled and tension is released, a greater desire follows. As desire continues to be fulfilled, a new and more intense desire is generated. In this way, through the gradual buildup and release of tension, she can feel her maximum desire for union and release it with an orgasm.

A secret of great sex is for the man to slowly tease a woman to increase her sexual desire. In the next chapter, we will explore the art of teasing.

CHAPTER 3

How to Increase a Woman's Pleasure

Women enjoy conversation most when they are not required to get to the point right away. Many times, to relax or to get closer to someone, they like to circle around for a while and gradually discover what they want to say. This is a perfect metaphor for how a woman enjoys sex. She loves it when a man takes time to get to the point and circles around for a while.

Until her desire and arousal is intense, a woman enjoys being touched in a nondirect manner. For example, before moving his fingers or the palms of his hands to touch her breasts, a man should circle them for a while, getting closer and closer. Then, when

he is about to touch, he should move somewhere else and start again.

Instead of being directly stimulated in her
most sensitive places, as a man likes, a
woman wants to be teased or gradually led
to the place where she is longing to be
touched. For example, when taking off her
bra, instead of just taking it off each time,
sometimes a man should slowly move his
finger along the inner lining, then slowly
pull down the bra strap, allowing the breast
to be exposed, and then cover it up again.

**A *woman wants to be teased or
gradually led to the place where
she is longing to be touched.***

A man can tease a woman by giving a little and then backing up to start over again.
Repeating this process generates more desire in her. Her increased longing provides
great pleasure for her as well as for him.

48

Once he realizes what is really turning her on, he begins to feel the power of restraining his own passion to drive her wild with pleasure.

〜 A Woman's Need to Relax

A man generally doesn't understand a woman's need to relax and get into sex slowly. He starts out ready to go. He does not readily understand a woman's need to relax first because sometimes he may want to have an orgasm so that he can relax. Unlike men, most women need to relax first before they can enjoy great sex.

Teasing and foreplay give her the time to relax and gradually let go of her inhibitions. Slow, rhythmic, and unpredictable physical touching, stroking, and rubbing of the nonerogenous zones gradually awaken a more intense longing to be touched in her erogenous zones. Before a man can fulfill a woman, she first needs time to relax and feel the part of her that needs to be filled up.

A piece of good advice commonly found in books about sex is for women to prepare for sex by taking a long warm bubble bath with the lights down low. Before I understood the differences between men and women, I could never understand this. If I took a long warm bath, I would probably fall asleep. Now, however, it makes sense to me that a woman could greatly benefit from a long warm bath.

Relaxation and gentle stimulation are the basis for a woman's arousal. By slowly tracing her body with his fingers and tender kisses, a man will awaken her more erogenous zones, which will long to be touched.

～ A Lover with a Slow Hand

When I interview women about what they want most from a man, again and again they tell me they want a lover with a slow hand. This slow process increases her pleasure so that when his fingers and tongue eventually move to touch her breasts, she is longing to be touched. When he moves to her inner thighs, she is already warm and ready to be touched. When she is stimulated in this way, her pleasure wells up from deep inside her being.

A man is different. Directly touching his penis dramatically increases his pleasure. Many women don't realize this and frustrate a man by waiting too long to touch him. If such touching seems too direct for her, a woman can relieve much of his frustration with the weight of her body pressing against his groin.

〜

A *woman needs to remember that direct stimulation provides maximum pleasure for a man.*

〜

Because men are different in this way, a man needs to practice going slow. When he

51

begins to consciously experience how wonderful it makes her feel, gradually it becomes more instinctive. A man needs to remember that to increase a woman's pleasure, he needs to delay direct stimulation. It will take longer and sometimes it will seem as if nothing is working, but eventually her pleasure will be much greater. If he takes this extra time, not only will she be happier, but he will also experience greater pleasure.

❧

A *man needs to remember that to increase a woman's pleasure, he needs to delay direct stimulation.*

❧

❧ Circumambulating the Temple

Certain ancient temples are dedicated to worshipping the female aspect of God. According to one ritual associated with these temples, you have to circumambulate the temple three times before entering it. This same principle applies to loving and adoring a woman during sex.

Before directly touching or entering a very delicate spot, a man should prepare her first. For example, when a man is kissing a woman, abruptly putting his tongue in her mouth can be too sudden. Instead, he should kiss her lightly several times, and then as she begins to open up, he can place his tongue in her mouth. One wonderful sensation is to first circle around inside her mouth before plunging more deeply.

When touching her breast, he should also circle first. For example, instead of directly touching her breast and then her nipple, he should first slowly move down toward the breast and then come back up. Then, with a slow rhythmic back and forth movement, he can get closer.

Once he begins to touch her breast, he can gracefully move his hand back and forth, cupping his hand around her breast in much the way her bra would. He could move his hand back and forth in a gentle rocking motion. Eventually, he can move all around the breast. Then he may squeeze and release it again and again. All these motions are designed to slowly and repetitively increase and then decrease stimulation.

One little tip that any man can easily learn is the art of taking off her bra. Years ago when I would take off my partner's bra, I would practically wrestle with the fasteners. Sex suddenly became very clumsy and awkward. How is a guy supposed to know how to take off a bra when he doesn't wear one?

This problem can be easily solved. One day when your wife is not around, find her bra drawer and take five minutes to examine her different bras. In a few minutes, you can become an expert. There are basically three kinds of fasteners: the up and down kind, the back and forth ones, and the ones in the front. Practice opening them so you can do it effortlessly with one hand. Then, with your eyes closed, practice doing it with one hand.

How to Increase a Woman's Pleasure

∽

The next time you have sex, she will be greatly impressed as you coolly and confidently release her bra. Women like men to have confidence. This is one area in which a man can definitely know what to do. As he releases her bra with one hand, she will begin to melt and surrender to his knowledgeable and masterful touch.

∽ How to Increase Desire

To increase her desire, a man may choose to touch her somewhere else and then come back to her breast and start all over. When he comes back this time, he may choose to get closer to the nipple. Instead of going directly, he should graze over it as if his touch is unintentional. This gives her a chance to feel her nipple's sensitivity and long for more.

When he comes back, he should circle the breast for a while. In this case, circling three times is not enough. Ten times longer than he would normally wait will probably do the trick.

Once he is touching the nipple, he can gently stroke it back and forth, back and forth, back and forth. The approach should be as though he has all the time in the world. Once he has touched the nipple, he can gently kiss or lick it.

Taking Off Her Panties

A man should begin to touch between her legs only when he thinks she is ready. Sometimes it is good to first touch around the lining of her panties and gradually explore her vulva.

It is very exciting for her if he doesn't just suddenly pull down her panties. Instead, he may start to pull them down and then pull them back up a little higher.

Instead of taking them off, he can begin touching her on the inside edge of her panties across the back, then the front, then along the edge down the front. Then he can put his fingers inside the edge between her legs.

Once he has checked with a gentle probing finger that she is moist, he can take off her panties. Or, instead of immediately pulling them off, he can once again delay pulling them down to convey the message that he is in control of his passions.

Even if his passion is mounting, he can take a long time. This restraint and control allow her to feel freer to release her inhibitions and let go of control. Instead of taking off her panties, he can reach around her buttocks and expose her bare bottom. He can begin to touch and stroke her buttocks and her inner thigh from behind.

Eventually, he can take off her panties and begin stroking her inner thighs and circling her whole vulva.

∽ Touching Her

Many times men forget to touch her most sensitive spot, the clitoris. In my counseling, I've often heard a woman complain that her partner doesn't touch her there, or that when he tries to, he misses the spot much of the time, or that even when he gets it right, he doesn't stay long enough. Many women see this as a sign that he doesn't really care about her.

That judgment is generally not true. A man forgets to touch her there because he doesn't instinctively understand how important it is. Here are some findings that will help a man to remember. In my own interviews and in most sexual studies; women report that ninety-eight percent of the orgasms they experience are directly the result of stimulation of the clitoris.

∽

∽

A man forgets to touch the clitoris not because he doesn't care about her fulfillment, but because he doesn't instinctively understand that almost all female orgasms result from the stimulation of her clitoris.

∽

Men, imagine having sex without having your penis stimulated. It would certainly not be very much fun. In a similar way, for a woman to enjoy great sex, stimulation of the clitoris for five to fifteen minutes is necessary if he wants her to have an orgasm.

Quite commonly in counseling, a man will tell me he touches his wife's clitoris for five or ten minutes. His wife, however, will privately tell me he rarely touches her there, and when he does, it is only for a minute or two.

I assure her that he really thinks he is taking more time and then teach her advanced skills for getting what she wants. By first accepting a man's tendencies to forget her needs, a woman can begin to get what she wants. If she is angry with him, it is hard for him to hear her legitimate requests.

∽ Taking More Time for Her

If a man is not touching a woman's clitoris for a long enough time, I suggest that she reach down and continue touching herself. In this way, he gets the message loud and clear but doesn't feel criticized, corrected, or controlled. When he experiences how much she is enjoying it, he will then automatically begin taking more time for her.

When there is another way she would like him to touch her, instead of patiently and silently bearing what he is doing, she can reach down and make the moves on herself that she wants him to make. At those times, the man should grab a pillow and go down there to watch and learn.

One very effective way a man can learn to give a woman a longer interlude in sex is to time it. It doesn't sound romantic, but it sure works. I recommend that the man discreetly put a clock by the bed. While he is touching her, he can occasionally glance over and time himself.

Men are often surprised to discover that when they are aroused, they truly are living in a different time zone. What feels like ten or fifteen minutes of stimulation is really only one or two minutes by the clock.

By setting himself up to take a full five to fifteen minutes, he can begin to give her the stimulation she really needs. When she is prepared in this way, she can more fully receive him when they begin intercourse.

∽ **Skillful Stimulation**

A skillful female lover directly stimulates a man's most sensitive and erogenous area. As these areas are stimulated, the rest of his body gradually wakes up and wants to be touched and stimulated as well. She can then successfully begin to use on him all the teasing techniques that would excite her. The trick with a man is to first stimulate his most pressing and sensitive organ.

A skillful male lover first stimulates a woman's least sensitive and least erogenous areas. First he might touch her hair, kiss her lips without yet inserting his tongue, wrap his arms around her, touch her legs but not her inner thighs, touch her back, or touch her buttocks. Then he might gently press his body against her, up and down, rubbing her with his groin back and forth in a circular motion.

By gradually moving around her body or rhythmically going back and forth on a certain area next to an erogenous zone, he wakes up her more sensitive areas and makes them want to be touched. Then, again in an indirect fashion, he can approach her more sensitive areas to provide repetitive stimulation.

〜

〜

A skillful male lover first stimulates a woman's least sensitive and least erogenous areas. A skillful female lover first stimulates a man's most pressing and sensitive organ.

〜

By mastering the art of slowly increasing her desire, a man can be confident that he knows what to do to drive his partner wild with pleasure. This confidence alone is very exciting to a woman. In the next chapter, we will explore how to increase sexual confidence.

CHAPTER 4

Sexual Confidence

Sexual confidence is the ultimate turn-on for both men and women. A woman is turned on when she feels her partner is confident that he knows how to fulfill her. His confidence assures her that he knows what to do, can be flexible if something isn't working, and has staying power. A man is turned on when a woman has confidence as well, but in a different way.

Sexual confidence is the ultimate turn-on.

When he senses her confidence in him, he is even more turned on. When her eyes give the message that she feels assured that she is going to have a good time, that he can do no wrong, and that she wants him to make love to her, he is very excited.

If a woman seems too confident that she knows what to do, it can possibly be intimidating. He may begin to wonder if he can do as much for her; he may begin to doubt that he can last long enough to satisfy her. Certainly, it is good for her to be confident in her abilities to satisfy him, but as with all advanced relationship skills, her greatest ability to fulfill him is through helping him be successful in fulfilling her.

∽

A *woman's* greatest ability to fulfill a man in sex is through helping him be successful in fulfilling her.

∽

∽ **Learning About Sex**

Before I began teaching seminars on sex, I had been a celibate monk for nine years. As a monk, I had been a teacher of spiritual philosophy and meditation. When I reached the age of twenty-seven, my life radically changed. I ceased being a monk, returned to the world, and started having sex again.

For the first year after nine years of abstinence, I was like a hungry man eating after a long fast. I felt a great need to make up for what I had missed. All I could think about was women, love, and sex. I had sex for breakfast, lunch, and dinner.

I read all I could about sex and had as much sex as possible. I wanted to learn as much as I could. Eventually, I began a Ph.D. program in sex and psychology.

When I was with a woman, I would explain to her that I had been a monk for nine years and was just learning about sex. I would ask her to teach me about her body and tell me what made her sexual experience the most fulfilling.

This approach had a tremendous effect. Somehow, women didn't mind my not knowing about sex because I had been a monk. Not only would they get really turned on telling me about what they liked in sex, but I really learned a lot.

After about two years of intense sexual experimentation according to various ancient traditions of the world, my sexual partner at the time and I started teaching workshops on sex and spirituality. Together we facilitated discussions about what made sex great for both men and women. Throughout the seminar, many participants talked openly about what made sex memorable.

Everyone benefited from this process of talking about male and female likes and dislikes. Although I was leading the discussions, I was clearly a student as well. I was taking notes and then trying things out with my partner at home.

∽ Why Talking Doesn't Always Work

Most men have never been monks and thus feel uncomfortable asking a woman the details of what she likes in sex. Not only does a man think he should already be a sexual expert, but a woman also wants her man to know what he is doing. She expects him to know intuitively what to do. She may also resist telling him what she likes because she doesn't want sex to be a pat formula but something they discover together.

Secretly, a woman may feel that if he is the right man or if he really loves her, he will know what to do. These feelings are food for romantic fantasy, but they don't create great sex. In addition, a woman is commonly afraid to let her wishes be known for fear that she may be judged in some way or that her partner won't do what she wants. For a variety of reasons, it just takes some of the romance out of sex if she has to tell him what to do.

∽

**Secretly, a woman may feel that if he is
the right man or if he really loves her,
he will know what to do. These feelings
are food for romantic fantasy, but they
don't create great sex.**

∽

While most books on sexuality say that it
is important to talk about sexual likes and
dislikes, couples generally don't do it. People in our society commonly are very inhibited when it comes to talking about sex, so
we generally only discuss sex when it is not
working. A partner who is dissatisfied begins to talk about what he or she wants, but
by then the other partner has trouble hearing about these needs. Instead of talking being a fun experience, it sounds like criticism
or blame, and usually to some degree it is.

Men are particularly sensitive about hearing feedback. When a woman tells him what
she would like or doesn't like, he hears her

saying, "You are not good enough. Other men know how to do it, why don't you? What's wrong with you?"

Ironically, a man is expected to know about sex, and because he is supposed to know, he can't ask her questions about what she likes and take time to learn about her. Just as women sometimes feel a need to fake orgasm to please him, men have to fake confidence to please her. Many men want to know more but don't know how to talk about sex without sounding as if they don't know all about it.

∽

Just as women sometimes feel a need to fake orgasm to please him, men have to fake confidence to please her.

∽

✎ Easy Ways to Talk About Sex

One way to overcome this lack of communication is to read books together that describe sex and then discuss them. It is a lot
easier to approach the subject of sex if your
partner doesn't feel blamed for doing it
wrong. When you hear something that feels
good to you, responding to it with a little
"ummm" or a bigger "ummm" gives your
partner the hint or reminder he or she needs.

No matter how much we know about sex,
understanding differences between men
and women adds a whole new slant. We are
much more motivated to give our partners
what they need when we understand the
differences.

Sometimes when I speak about sex, I ask
my audience to clap when they really like
what I am saying, to emphasize to their partners that the point I am making rings true
for them. Men are surprised at the times
when the women clap the hardest, and vice
versa. A husband doesn't take it so personally when his wife claps because almost all

the women are clapping, and besides, she is just clapping at what she likes, not complaining about him. She doesn't need to tell him directly what she needs because he can observe her reaction.

Through directly experiencing feedback in this nonthreatening way, many couples who had even stopped having sex suddenly started to enjoy great sex. By learning about their differences in this way, men and women are more able to remember them and are thus more motivated to do what it takes to create great sex for themselves and their partners.

∽ Every Woman Is Different

Not only are men and women different, but every woman is different. For a man to truly understand what a woman needs, a simple discussion at some point can make a big and lasting difference. To complicate matters more, not only are women different, but over time they change and then may change back. While general techniques and approaches can be discussed in a book or seminar, your partner's unique preferences cannot.

∽

Every woman is different. For a man to truly understand what she needs, a simple discussion at some point can make a big and lasting difference.

∽

For Sam, touching a woman's most sensitive zone was a hit-or-miss process. When she was getting all aroused, he knew he was doing something right, but didn't exactly know what. So that he could become more confident, I suggested that he ask his partner, Ellen, to take a few minutes to teach him about her body. I recommended that they talk about it in a casual and detached manner without trying to get turned on.

In a very matter-of-fact way rather than

some sexy conversation, she explained briefly what she liked most. At first, Ellen was a little shy about it, but Sam assured her that it would really help. Years later, Sam can still remember every word she said.

With a clear understanding of what a woman likes most, a man can relax. While he doesn't have to be mechanical about it and follow her suggestions to the letter every time they make love, an awareness of her preferences gives him the confidence to create a new sexual experience each time. When something does not seem to be working, he knows he can always come back to what she likes the most. This kind of confidence helps a man to relax in sex and actually be more creative and sponta-neous.

❧

A man feels free to try new things when he knows he can always come back to the tried and true.

❧

∽ The Book of Love

In response to Sam's request, Ellen said, "You want the book on how to make love to me?" Sam smiled and agreed.

In the privacy of their bedroom, Ellen first talked for a while about some of the ways she liked to be touched and where. He then asked her to show him how she liked to be touched between the legs. In a kind of clinical way, she began to show him. She was not really trying to stimulate herself but was just showing him her favorite moves.

After watching for a while, Sam looked very closely and repeated her moves just to get them right. He tried to remember clearly what her vulva looked like when she touched herself so that he could make the same motions with the same accuracy without looking.

To practice, they used a mirror. He lay down beside her and reached down to her vulva and began touching her with one hand while holding the mirror with the other hand. As he touched her genitals, he also watched his movements in the mirror. Later, when they were really having sex and she was moaning with excitement, he knew what was pleasing her because he could clearly visualize what his hands were doing and where they were touching.

During their talk, Sam carefully studied the terrain of her sexual organs, particularly the clitoris. Because he knew precisely what she looked like, Ellen was assured of always getting the stimulation she needed, but most importantly, Sam knew exactly what he was doing.

While this worked wonders to improve their sex life, I also suggested to Sam that when sex was exceptionally great, he could again ask Ellen what she liked most. At those times, I explained to Ellen, she should be careful to focus on what she liked so as not to sound critical.

If Sam asked specifically about something and she didn't like it, instead of going into great detail, I told Ellen, she should just pause for a while as if to say she was thinking of a nice way to say that she didn't like it. This consideration makes negative feedback much easier to hear.

Sometimes she might say, "It was nice," or "It was all right," but without much enthusiasm. Sam would get the clear message that it didn't go over big. If something was displeasing to her, she might say, "I'm not really into that." These kind, gentle comments make it easy for Sam to ask again in the future.

By asking her from time to time what she likes, Sam allows her to share any new discoveries or shifts in her awareness of what she likes in sex. Likewise, Sam would almost always let her know when she did something that he really liked.

∽ When to Talk About Sex

It is just not romantic to ask a woman what she wants while you are having sex. It is best done either after sex or at another time when you are not immediately planning to have sex. During sex, she doesn't want to think about her needs; instead, she wants to *feel* more and let it all gradually unfold.

To gather information about what a woman likes in bed, a man should listen carefully to how she responds during sex. A man needs to hear a woman verbally express her pleasure. That way, he gets the feedback he needs to know what is working to fulfill her. A woman may even enjoy sex more when she expresses her feelings verbally.

To get more direct feedback, a man can ask, but ideally he should do it when it seems as if sex has been rather good. Another good time to ask is in response to a comment in a book you are reading, or a lecture or movie scene.

This kind of conversation needs to be casual and not too direct. For example, a man should not take notes and then say, "OK, first you want this and then you want that, then after this I should do that."

This approach is too mechanical for her.

She needs to feel that when he is having sex with her, he is expressing his feelings and not following a formula.

∽ Giving Hot and Cold Feedback During Sex

Men are particularly sensitive about sexual feedback. When a man hears a woman's suggestions or requests, sometimes he feels he is being corrected or criticized, and this is hard for many men to handle.

Giving "hot" and "cold" messages can help your partner tremendously. At some time in your life, you have probably played the game of finding something that was hidden. The way to help the person looking, without directly telling, was to give hot and cold messages.

When the searcher was getting closer you'd say, "Warmer," and when the searcher was getting farther away, you would say, "Cooler." In a similar fashion, a woman can make sounds during sex that say, "You are getting warmer," or sounds that say, "You are getting cooler."

These responses are very important. It is as though he is wearing a blindfold and needs her responses to find his way. With every touch, he needs to know whether it is hot or cold. Feedback is very important for him to learn about her body over time.

Sometimes a woman may be enjoying the relaxing phase of sex, and making no sounds is a natural expression of her inner calm and relaxation. This is confusing because at other times, no sounds could mean he is not stimulating her the right way and she is not getting into it. The solution is for her to verbally let him know if she is quietly enjoying the relaxation.

She could say, "This feels so good. I like just cuddling for a while," or "It feels so good to just relax for a while and enjoy your touch," or simply, "Umm, I like this." This will give him the patience and understanding he needs to proceed.

✑ How to Give Positive Direction

When a man is doing something that is uncomfortable for her or that she doesn't want, the best technique is to move him in the direction that will be more pleasurable. As with other advanced relationship skills, the approach that works best is to help him be successful rather than focus on his mistakes.

In sex, she can just move his hand where she would like it and make a pleasurable response. He will quickly get the message. For example, if she wants to verbally say something, she should ideally say, "I like this," instead of "I don't like that."

✑ Ten Sexual Turnoffs

When a woman doesn't understand a man's sensitivities in this area, she will tend to unintentionally turn him off by saying things like this:

1. "You're not doing it right."
2. "I don't like that."
3. "Ouch! That hurts!"
4. "Don't touch me like that."
5. "That tickles."
6. "Not like that."
7. "Not yet."
8. "Not there."
9. "I'm not ready."
10. "What are you doing?"

This kind of feedback can simply shut a man off immediately. One minute he is aroused, and the next he is not.

∽ **Why a Man Shuts Down**

Many times during sex, a man's one goal is to please his partner. At those times, he is more sensitive to negative feedback. If he makes a mistake and feels criticized, sometimes the only thing a woman can do is accept that his feelings have been hurt and he just needs a little time before he can become aroused again.

∽

When a man is seeking to please his partner, he is most sensitive to negative feedback.

∽

Here's an example of how a woman can unintentionally cause a man to shut down. During sex with Jake, Annie kept saying things like, "Not like that," "I don't like that," and "That tickles." Well, after three strikes, Jake was out. Suddenly, he stopped. In an instant, all his feelings were gone. He lost all his attraction to her and was simply turned off.

She said, "What's wrong?"

He didn't answer.

After waiting a few moments, she said, "Weren't we just having sex?"

He said, "Yes."

She said, "Well, are we going to continue having sex?"

He said, "No," and then rolled over and went to sleep.

In counseling, I advised Jake to discuss with Annie what had happened. He told her, "During sex, I think I am very sensitive to certain comments. I would rather you move my hand where you want it than tell me you don't like it. If I am tickling you, then I would rather you just pull my hand away and try not to laugh, particularly if I happen to be in a serious mood. If my touch tickles, you could also just apply pressure to my fingers to give me a message to press harder and not continue tickling you with a feather touch."

To Jake's surprise, Annie was very open to his comments, and he greatly appreciated that. Afterward, when Annie occasionally would say something that he felt was a turnoff, Jake did his best to dodge and let it pass.

Even if a man's arousal goes away for a little while, if he just pretends that everything is fine, with a little time it comes back. To stop and discuss why he shut down is generally not effective in returning him to a state of arousal.

᭒

Even if a man's arousal goes away for a little while, if he just pretends that everything is fine, with a little time it comes back.

᭒

᭒ **Sounds Verses Sentences**

To give feedback in sex, it is best for women to make little noises and not use complete sentences. When a woman uses complete sentences, it can be a turnoff. Using complete sentences is a subtle clue to him that she is still in her head and not fully in her body.

Sometimes a woman will say things she read in a romance novel, such as "Your touch makes me long for you to enter my body." To a man, this can sound stilted. It just doesn't sound as if it's coming from her feelings. To give him the same message much more effectively, she can make deep sounds like "uumph" or high sounds like "ohhh." A woman's feeling responses to a man's touch give him all the feedback he needs.

᛫

A *woman's responses* to a man's touch give him all the feedback he needs.

᛫

If a woman is using complete sentences, it may be because she is turned on when a man uses them. It is very impressive to a woman when a man can be aroused and also talk to her.

A man tends to be silent as his arousal is building. Although he has the ability to talk in complete sentences, he doesn't do it; he doesn't like her to talk in complete sentences and so he doesn't realize that she will love it.

Talking to her in complete sentences not only increases her arousal but can raise her self-esteem and help her to love her body.

∽ Twenty Sexual Turn-on Phrases

These are some phrases he can use to increase her pleasure if they express his true feelings. He should not use these phrases just to turn her on. It is important that they be genuine expressions of what is true inside him that perhaps he didn't realize were important to say. Here is a list of twenty:

1. "You are so beautiful."
2. "You are my dream come true."
3. "I love you so much."
4. "I love sharing my life with you."
5. "You turn me on so much."

6. "Your breasts turn me on."
7. "I love touching your soft skin."
8. "I love holding you in my arms."
9. "I love your breasts."
10. "I love your legs."
11. "Your breasts are perfect."
12. "Your lips are perfect."
13. "You feel so good."
14. "You feel so hot."
15. "You are so delicious."
16. "You are so sexy."
17. "I am all yours."
18. "All my love is for you."
19. "I love having sex with you."
20. "I long for you."

These messages clearly expressed or whispered in her ear help her to feel loved, which in turn opens her up to her more intense sexual desires. With all the media and magazines focusing on women with perfect bodies, it is difficult for a woman to accept that her partner truly adores her body.

I always get lots of applause from women when I recount this list of things to say. The comments about the breasts especially get big applause. Men don't realize that women love and need to hear such things again and again. A man will feel during sex that his partner's breasts are perfect, but he doesn't realize that she needs to hear it. He mistakenly thinks it is enough that he wants to touch them.

The manager of a women's lingerie store told me this story. While a group of women over age sixty were shopping, one of them was trying on a very sexy outfit. The other women were shaking their heads and telling her that she couldn't wear it. With great confidence, she responded, "When you are the only naked woman in the room, to him you are a million dollars." This comment revealed an insight that most women do not know about men. When a man loves you, the more aroused he becomes, the more perfect your body becomes to him. The last thing on a man's mind during sex is how fat your thighs are.

∽

**When you are the only naked woman
in the room, to him you are a
million dollars.**

∽

∽ When Men Look at Other Women

When every man's head turns in a trance as a woman with a "10" body walks by, all the other women in the room are reminded that they don't have "10" bodies. This can be hard on a woman's self-image. Expressing love to a woman using complete sentences when she is open and naked in his arms not only arouses her but also helps her to feel really good about herself and grateful to be with such a loving man.

∾

When every man's head turns in a trance as a woman with a "10" body walks by, all the other women in the room are reminded that they don't have "10" bodies. This can be hard on a woman's self-image.

∾

A woman doesn't instinctively understand that the same man who stares at the "10" body, when in love and turned on by her, is also totally entranced by the feminine beauty of her body, regardless of where the media would rank it on a scale of one to ten.

When a man loves a woman and she is expressing her femininity in their relationship, he is attracted to her, not just to her body. The more he is attracted to her, the more beautiful her body is to him. Attraction that is only skin deep cannot last a long time. Quite commonly, an attraction that is only physical is quickly burned out, like a match.

∽ Men Are Attracted Visually

It is important for women to understand that
men are first attracted to a woman visually.
A man sees a beautiful woman and instinctively wants to look at her body. When a
woman sees a handsome man, she may
want to get to know him but not just because
of his looks. She is not immediately concerned about his body.

A woman commonly misunderstands and
assumes that a man is superficial if he is attracted primarily to the physical. She does
not realize that he too wants to get to know
her, but the place he starts is the body.

At first, men are most turned on visually
while a woman is most interested in getting
to know the person. Gradually, as the relationship unfolds, a man becomes more and
more turned on to the inner person. As a
woman loves the inner man gradually over
time, she is increasingly attracted and
turned on to his body as well.

Even if at times in the beginning of a relationship a man is not sure he is fully satisfied

with his partner's body, over time, as he grows to know her and love her, he will begin to experience the perfection of her body for him. It is quite easy for a single man to be hypnotized by the media about what makes a woman beautiful. He compares a woman to what he sees on TV and in magazines. Fortunately, when he is aroused and growing in love with a woman, the spell of the media is broken, and he can fully appreciate her beauty.

At these times in sex, he should reassure her by saying sweet nothings about how beautiful her body is to him. This not only frees him from the influence of the media but frees her as well.

〜 **A Simple Solution**

Without an awareness of how men are attracted visually, a woman begins to feel unattractive when her partner looks at another woman, and begins to resent him as well. The solution to this problem can be simple.

A woman needs to accept a man's natural visual appreciation of other women, and when a man looks, he needs to look appropriately. Once Bonnie and I were in an elevator with another older couple and a nineteen-year-old female model in a string bikini. This time, it was even difficult for the women not to look. When we got out of the elevator, the other woman said to her husband, "George, it's OK to look, but don't drool!"

〜

A *woman needs to accept a man's natural visual appreciation of other women, and when a man looks, he needs to look appropriately.*

〜

Appropriateness and a sensitivity to your partner's feelings is the answer. When I happen to notice another woman and enjoy looking at her, I will out of consideration for my wife turn back around and give her some special attention. It is my way of saying, "Yes, that was a beautiful woman. Oh, how I like beautiful women. I am such a lucky guy to be married to such a beautiful woman. You are the one I want to be with."

By turning back to her and being a little affectionate, I assure her that she is the one I want to be with. Instead of being turned off, she is able to warm up to me instead.

⌁ Time, Time, and More Time

If we want confidence to grow and passion to last over time, we must take more time in sex. While a man may need only a few minutes of stimulation to have an orgasm, a woman generally needs much more. With this understanding, a man can remain confident that he is doing the right things even though his partner is taking much longer to become aroused.

Timing is one of the biggest sexual differences between men and women. A man is biologically wired to become fully aroused very quickly, like a blowtorch, while a woman is wired to become aroused slowly and gradually.

∽ How Much Time?

Basically, a man needs about two or three minutes of stimulation to have an orgasm. It is generally a very simple process, as easy as shaking up a can of beer and then letting it pop!

A woman generally needs about ten times that amount of time. She needs twenty to thirty minutes of foreplay and stimulation.

If a man wants to give a woman an orgasm, he should remember this: For her to experience the big "O," he needs to place the "O" after his two to three minutes, making it twenty to thirty minutes.

∽

**For a woman to experience the big "O,"
a man needs to place the "O" after his
two to three minutes, making it twenty
to thirty minutes.**

∽

Many times a man will be done after a few
minutes and truly assume that she was just
as happy and fulfilled.

He says, "Are you satisfied?"

She feels like saying, "Not even close."

∽ Sexual Versus Emotional Fulfillment

Intercourse feels so good to him, he can't
imagine that it wasn't as wonderful for her.
When she tells him that she didn't have an
orgasm, he is easily confused or frustrated.
Without understanding that she needs ten

times more time than he does, he can easily feel powerless to turn her on.

During intercourse, she may also be making noises of pleasure and fulfillment. This does not always mean that she is getting the stimulation she needs. Many times the pleasure she feels is her emotional response to his pleasure. It feels good to connect to him emotionally and provide him with such pleasure, and it increases her desire, but emotional fulfillment does not stimulate her sexually. She needs the touch and the time if she is to have the orgasm.

༚

Emotional fulfillment is not enough.
A woman needs touch and more time
if she is to have the orgasm.

༚

In real estate, there is a saying to help us understand the value of a property: "Location, location, location." In sex, it is "Time, time, and more time."

When a woman gets the time she needs, she can feel confident that she will get the fulfillment she is looking for. When a man understands that it is not so much what he does but how long he takes to do it that makes the difference, his confidence is also increased.

A man instinctively feels confident when his partner has regular orgasms. If she doesn't have an orgasm each time, he begins to worry. In the next chapter, we will explore how sometimes a woman can be fulfilled in sex without having an orgasm.

CHAPTER 5

*W*omen Are Like the Moon, Men Are Like the Sun

Women are like the moon in that their sexual experience is always waxing or waning. Sometimes, regardless of what a great lover he is, she will not have an orgasm. She is not only unable to have an orgasm, but she may not even want one. This difference between men and women is very important for men to understand.

In her sexual cycle, which tends to last approximately twenty-eight days, sometimes she really wants an orgasm and her body is ripe and ready, while at other times she would rather cuddle and be close. She could have sex at these times and even be aroused, but her body doesn't care to have an orgasm.

❧

❧

Sometimes a woman really wants an orgasm and her body is ripe and ready, while at other times she would rather cuddle and be close.

❧

Sometimes she is in the full-moon stage of her cycle, sometimes she is in the half-moon stages, and sometimes she is in the new-moon stage. In each of these phases and all the many phases in between, her sexual longings will vary. There is no way to predict which stage she is in. Even from month to month, the length of the cycle varies.

Men do not instinctively understand this difference because they are not like the moon in this regard. Men are like the sun. Every morning, it rises with a big smile!

When a man gets turned on, his body generally wants a release. He wants his orgasm, and he is generally quite capable of having one. If he gets aroused and then doesn't have a release, not only will he feel emotionally dissatisfied, but he may also experience physical discomfort. This is why it is hard for him to imagine his partner not wanting or needing release every time she has sex. She may enjoy the closeness of sex but not want an orgasm. When she is not interested or doesn't have an orgasm, he mistakenly assumes something is wrong.

〜 How Men Measure Success in Sex

Men tend to measure their success in sex by a woman's orgasm. If she doesn't have one, he may pout for hours. This is why a woman feels pressured to perform in sex even if she doesn't feel like it. She may fake sexual pleasure just to satisfy him.

This pressure on her to perform prevents sex from being completely fulfilling for her. It also prevents her from experiencing the natural ebb and flow of her sexual experience. If she has to be equally responsive or orgasmic for him each time, she can't relax and discover where sex will naturally take her.

❧

Pressure on a woman to have an orgasm prevents sex from being completely fulfilling for her.

❧

Once a woman feels she has to fake orgasms or perform, it can prevent her from having real orgasms. It is said that many of the great "sex goddesses" as proclaimed by the media were actually nonorgasmic in their real personal relationships.

The pressure to have an orgasm each time can prevent a woman from having them at those times when her body really can have one. One of the requirements for great sex is that a woman not feel pressured to perform in any way. This can be easily accomplished through an understanding of how men and women are different.

A great sex life means that sometimes sex

will be a super fantastic memory never to be forgotten, while at other times it may not be so intense, but it is loving and both partners get what they want; the man gets his orgasm, and whether or not she's in the mood to have an orgasm, she gets the physical affection she wants.

〜 *Memorable Sex*

One time while getting undressed before bed, I looked over at my wife while she was also getting undressed. I suddenly began thinking about the possibility of having sex that night.

I said, "Did we have sex this morning?"

She smiled and said, "Yeah, it was real memorable, wasn't it?"

I laughed.

This exchange best describes for me the difference between regular sex and memorable sex. A great sex life includes both regular sex *and* regular memorable sex.

Although one may know the skills of memorable sex, it is easy to forget to use them and settle for a routine of regular sex. Men particularly forget how to create memorable sex. It is not that they don't care, but they just forget what is important to the woman.

Men are more driven to be efficient. When twenty minutes of foreplay works, a subconscious impulse emerges saying, "Let's see if ten minutes can create the same effect." Quite automatically, he forgets her need for *more* time.

⌒ **Why Men Forget**

Having a great sex life doesn't mean you experience fireworks every time, but it does require you to persist in being aware of your partner's different needs. Ideally, each time both the man and the woman should feel they are getting what they need.

Men commonly tend to forget what a

110

woman needs to be fulfilled in sex. In the beginning, he may go very slow in sex because he is not sure of what she likes or he is not sure that she is willing to let him touch her. But once they are having sex regularly, he doesn't realize that it was his slow and tentative movements that were so arousing to her. Even when a man has read about these differences, because they are not his instinctive experience, he may easily forget them in the heat of his passion.

~

Once they are having sex regularly,
a man doesn't realize that it was
his slow and tentative movements
that were so arousing to her.

~

Commonly, a woman will feel as if he doesn't care about her. Even if a man cares deeply, he can still forget and not even know he is forgetting. I remember a surprising experience in the first year of our marriage. After giving an evening lecture on sex, while driving home I asked Bonnie if she had liked my talk.

She said, "I love hearing you talk about sex. That's why I always come to your sex lectures. You describe it so clearly."

I said rather proudly and confidently, "When I describe great sex, is that what I do?" I was expecting her to say, "Oh yes."

Instead, she hesitantly said, "Well . . . you used to do it more."

I said, "You mean I don't do all those things?"

She said, "Well, recently you've kind of been in a hurry."

I said, "Well, tonight we will have lots of time."

She said, "Ummm, that sounds good."

Her noncritical tone of voice helped me not to feel defensive. I share this story to make the point that even when I regularly used to teach audiences about great sex, I could forget the very basics of taking more time for her.

When a man doesn't take the time a woman needs, one skill for slowing him down is to make a brief, well-chosen comment like this:

"Oh, this feels so good. Let's go real slow."

"Let's make sure we have plenty of time."

"Tonight I want to take a long time."

These kinds of comments are informative but not corrective or controlling.

∽ What Makes Sex Memorable

While listening to men and women share stories of memorable sex in my early seminars, I began to notice a common theme. A man would tell stories about how a woman responded to him. He was proud of how he had taken her to higher states of ecstasy.

Women, on the other hand, described more how they felt and what he did for her. The buildup was more important to her than the end result. Women would proudly describe what the man did to provide for her fulfillment. This different theme is very significant.

The bottom line of what makes sex fulfilling and memorable for a man is a woman's fulfillment. When a man is successful in fulfilling her, he feels most fulfilled.

∽

**What makes sex fulfilling
and memorable for a man
is a woman's fulfillment.**

∽

What makes sex fulfilling and memorable for a woman is the same, her fulfillment. Certainly, she wants him to be fulfilled, but his fulfillment is not a primary cause of her pleasure. It doesn't give her the physical stimulation she needs for orgasm. Women do not commonly say things like, "Sex was really great because he had such a great orgasm." When a man is successful in fulfilling her, sex is great for her.

For sex to be memorable from both the male and female perspectives, the woman needs to be fulfilled. I have never heard a man complain, "She had a great time and I didn't. All she cared about was herself and her own pleasure. She had her way with me and then left."

When Her Pleasure Becomes His Pleasure

The more emotionally connected to a woman a man is, the more her pleasure becomes his pleasure. Through connecting with her physically, he can also connect with her emotionally and can actually experience her fulfillment as his own.

If a woman has a great time, the man

tends to take credit, and it excites him even more. His fulfillment and pleasure are ensured by her fulfillment. As we have discussed, his fulfillment in sex is determined or measured by her maximum fulfillment. If she doesn't have an orgasm, he mistakenly thinks that she was not fulfilled. This tendency can be overcome when he understands that she can be just as fulfilled without always having an orgasm.

❧

Sometimes a woman can be just as fulfilled without having an orgasm.

❧

It is such a relief for both partners when the man finally understands that a woman can be fulfilled sometimes without an orgasm. He can stop measuring the success of sex by whether she had an orgasm, and she can stop feeling the pressure to have an orgasm when her body is not responding in that way. Instead, he can measure success by her fulfillment, and she can relax and enjoy the sex without the pressure. Men need to remember that women are like the moon and sometimes can be fulfilled even without an orgasm.

Women I've counseled have expressed this truth in different ways:

> "I don't need to have an orgasm each time. If I don't have an orgasm, it doesn't mean something is wrong."

> "Sometimes to be fulfilled, I just want to be held. I am happy if he has an orgasm, but I don't really want one. It is just not there. At other times, it is there and I definitely want to have one."

> "I like having orgasms sometimes, but at other times, what I like most is the touching and cuddling."

> "Sometimes sex is too much about get-
> ting to the orgasm. I find myself try-
> ing to have one, and all the fun is
> gone. I want it to be OK with him if I
> don't have one. It's OK with me."

When a man doesn't understand that
women are like the moon, it is not only very
frustrating for him, but also puts a lot of
pressure on women to perform.

🖂 Why Women Are Surprised

When I talk in groups about how men want
a woman to be fulfilled, it is clearly a surprise to most of the women. They feel in response, "If he is so concerned with my
fulfillment, then why is he in such a hurry to
fulfill his own passions?" With an understanding of how we are different, it becomes
easy to answer this question.

Men want a woman to be fulfilled but mistakenly assume that what makes him happy

makes her happy. Just as he is fulfilled through her pleasure, he assumes she will be just as happy with his pleasure. He does not instinctively know that she needs more time, nor does he realize all the other requirements that women have for great sex.

As I have mentioned repeatedly, a woman's sexual fulfillment is much more complex than a man's. She requires a man with a skillful touch, lots of time, and a loving attitude. For a man, once he is aroused, it is generally a given that he will have an orgasm.

His problem, which we will discuss a little later, is that he may have an orgasm too soon; from his side, she takes too long and from her side, he is too quick. This problem is easily solved as men begin to understand how to prolong the sexual experience to fulfill her basic needs. Once she is fulfilled, then at other times she can be more supportive of occasions when he doesn't want to take a long time.

Men and women are actually very compatible. For those times when a woman is like the full moon, needing an orgasm, a man can greatly enjoy taking her to higher levels of pleasure and fulfillment. At those times when she is a half-moon or less, her need to be touched can be fulfilled while he gets to enjoy sex freely without having to hold back. In the latter case he can quickly have an orgasm in a few minutes, the way he was biologically wired to.

Sometimes they can choose to take a long time so that she gets her orgasm, and at other times, when she is not in the mood for it, he can enjoy the unrestrained freedom of just going for his own. At these times, he is like a sprinter running to his goal. At other times, he is like a long distance runner and is required to pace himself to last as long as it takes.

When a Woman Doesn't Want an Orgasm

Sometimes when a woman begins sex, she doesn't know whether her body wants to have an orgasm or not. She doesn't know if she is in the full-moon or half-moon phase of her cycle. She may feel romanced by her partner and want to have sex, but as sex progresses, she may discover that her body doesn't want to have an orgasm.

When the man is taking a lot of time trying to give her an orgasm and she is trying to have one but her body is just not responding, it can be very frustrating to them both. He feels as if something is wrong and blames her or himself. Without understanding her moon phases, she may feel that something is wrong with her. She will try to perform and respond for him, but it is not real. This can minimize sexual confidence for them both and leave a disturbing memory that minimizes their desire to have sex.

Once both partners understand the woman's sexual cycle, these old frustrations disappear. Repeatedly, women tell me that by just hearing that they are like the moon, they are released to become orgasmic. A woman who has difficulty opening up in sex begins to open up when she doesn't feel the

121

pressure to have an orgasm. Not having to respond leads her to the place where her responses are more natural. By not trying to have an orgasm one day, she is freed to have an orgasm at another time.

∽

A *woman who has difficulty opening up in sex begins to open up when she doesn't feel the pressure to have an orgasm.*

∽

During sex, if a woman begins to realize that she is not going to have an orgasm, instead of continuing to try, she can say, "Let's just have a quickie." This little phrase can make a world of difference. He has no problem shifting from trying to give her an orgasm to suddenly concentrating on his own orgasm.

Her not having an orgasm is only difficult when they don't share an understanding that he has not failed her. When she says, "Let's just have a quickie," a part of him feels let off the hook. It reminds him that it is not his fault or hers; it is just not the time for her to have an orgasm. He can successfully fulfill her just by being affectionate and holding her while he climaxes.

Just as a man needs to take a long time for the woman to be fulfilled in sex, sometimes he needs her to not take a long time. In the next chapter, we will explore the joy of quickies for men, and women can be assured of getting what they need as well.

CHAPTER 6

The Joy of "Quickies"

While many books talk about taking time for the woman to have a pleasurable experience, none seem to talk about the man's legitimate need to *not* take a lot of time.

Although most men are happy to please their partners, sometimes a man can feel that he just wants to skip all the foreplay and, as the slogan goes, just do it. Something deep inside him wants to cut loose and completely let go without any restraint or worry about lasting longer or what he should do to make his partner happy. It's not that he doesn't want her to be happy, it's that he doesn't want to hold himself back.

To be patient and regularly take the time a woman needs in sex, a man needs to enjoy an occasional quickie. When he can follow his instincts once in a while to fulfill his need to "go for it" without all the buildup and foreplay, he can more easily take the time she needs on other occasions. Just as a car needs to run occasionally at high speeds on the highway to clean out the carburetor, some part of a man just needs to attain his sexual expression without any slowing down.

∽

To *be patient and regularly take the time a woman needs in sex, a man needs to enjoy an occasional quickie.*

∽

Feeling this need inside and acting on it are two different things. For example, even when James and Lucy did have quickies, James always felt a little guilty because it was clear that Lucy didn't get what she needed.

James felt that having sex without fore-play for her was selfish and he was not be-ing a good lover. To try to solve this problem, he would wait till he was almost late for work and then initiate sex with Lucy.

He would say, "Well, I only have a few minutes because I need to leave for work. Let's have sex before I go." She was very co-operative, and he would experience the joy of having a quickie guilt-free.

After a while, this didn't feel right. James didn't want to have to be late in order to en-joy an occasional quickie. To more effec-tively solve this problem, I suggested that James and Lucy negotiate.

❧ Quickies for Cuddles

James said to Lucy, "Sometimes I would just like to have sex without all the foreplay. I know it doesn't give you what you want, but it would sure feel good to me." I asked Lucy,

"What could James do to support you so that you would feel good about supporting him with quickies?"

She said, "I'm not sure. I guess I have a lot of considerations. I'm worried that if I willingly have quickies with James, that's all I will get."

He said, "OK, that makes sense. What if I promise to have more leisurely sex with you just as much as we are having now?"

She said, "That's good. What about really special sex or a romantic getaway for an evening at least once a month?"

James agreed. In return for an occasional quickie, or "fast food sex," they would have leisurely or "healthy home-cooked sex" once or twice a week, and at least once a month they would schedule a special time with no interruptions for "gourmet sex." I asked Lucy, "Is there anything else you need James to do so that you will be comfortable indulging him in quickies?"

She said, "It all sounds great, but I still don't feel completely comfortable with the idea of quick sex." She turned to James and said, "When we have a quickie, it is sometimes over in three or four minutes. By the time you are done, I am just getting started. I feel like you expect me to be all excited and responsive. I can't in that short time period."

James said, "That's OK. I can give that to you. If you are OK with occasional quickies, I promise to never expect you to respond. It will just be your gift to me. I don't expect you to get anything out of it."

She laughed and said, "OK, but there is more." Lucy realized that in this moment she had great negotiating power. She had the moon and she was going for the stars as well, and James was glad to go with her.

She said, "If you are going to have regular quickies, then I want cuddles. I want to feel your willingness to cuddle with me for a few minutes without you necessarily wanting sex."

He said, "No problem. Just tell me that you want to cuddle and that's it. I'll restrain

myself and just be warm and affectionate."
He paused. "Is that it?"

She said, "I think that's it."

The Four Conditions

I thought this was a terrific deal, and so did
James and Lucy. To make sure that their
quickies would be guilt-free, I suggested
that they summarize their deal.

James said to Lucy, "So given these four
conditions: regular healthy home-cooked
sex, gourmet sex once a month, no expectations during the quickie, and regular cuddles, you will then be happy to have fast
food sex with me."

She said, "It sounds good. But still if I'm
just too tired or not feeling up to it for whatever reason, I don't want to feel like I have
to say yes."

James happily agreed.

〜

〜 How to Increase Sexual Attraction

This new deal completely improved James and Lucy's sex life in ways that they couldn't imagine. James's sexual attraction for Lucy began to increase dramatically.

James described it this way: "For the first time in my sexual history, I felt completely free. I was suddenly free to skip foreplay and go right to intercourse. For the first time, I was not at all concerned about my performance or having to please. It was strictly for me, and there was no sinking guilty feeling that she wasn't getting what she needed. We both feel good about it because we know she will get hers at another time."

For James and most men, the freedom to have guilt-free quickies is as liberating as going into a store and knowing that you can buy anything you want, or being able to drive your car without any speed limits; it is like riding a motorcycle without having to wear a helmet. It is definitely a very adolescent feeling, but it also brings new life into a man's life and into the relationship. After all, it is in adolescence that a young man is in his sexual prime. No wonder this newfound sexual freedom greatly recharges a man's sex life.

In addition, after James and Lucy made this agreement, he was never hesitant to initiate sex because there was no possibility of feeling rejected. On most occasions, when he initiated sex, if she was not in the mood, instead of saying no, which would make him feel rejected, she would simply say yes to a quickie.

Interestingly, after a few years of guilt-free quickies, they were not so important to James. Many times when he initiates sex and she is not in the mood, rather than have a quickie, he will happily wait until she too wants sex.

Knowing that he can almost always have a quickie and that she is happy to give him one, when she is not in the mood for more leisurely sex, he doesn't feel in the slightest way rejected. This feeling that he will not be rejected is essential for a man to continue to be passionately attracted to his partner. Once this agreement is made and the man doesn't feel rejected, it is still a great feeling for a man just to go for it sometimes without having to put on the brakes.

How to Safely Initiate Sex Even When She's Not in the Mood

By making quickies guilt-free, a woman automatically supports a man in feeling free to initiate sex. These are some common phrases for initiating sex and common answers a woman can give instead of just saying no.

1. He says, "I'm feeling really turned on to you. Let's have sex."	She says, "I'm not in the mood for sex, but we could have a quickie."

2. He says, "I've missed you. Let's find some time to have sex."

She says, "Um, that sounds like a good idea. I don't have a lot of time right now, but we could have a quickie."

3. He says, "I have some time. Would you like to have sex?"

She says, "We could have a quickie now and then maybe tomorrow we could schedule more time to have sex."

4. He says, "Would you like to go upstairs and spend some intimate time together?"

She says, "We could have a quickie. Maybe that will help me relax a little, and then we could talk."

5. He says, "Let's schedule some time today to make love."

She says, "Well, I'm not in the mood for a lot of foreplay, but a quickie would be nice. Sometimes I like the closeness of sex even though I don't feel like an orgasm."

6. He says, "I'm feeling so turned on. I would love to have sex."

She says, "I would love that too. We don't have much time, so why don't we have a quickie?"

7. He says, "Let's have sex tonight."

She says, "I've really got a bad headache. Maybe we could have sex tomorrow. We could have a quickie right now."

8. He says nothing but gently reaches over in bed and begins making the moves.

She whispers, "Um, this feels good. Don't worry about me tonight. Just go for it."

9. They are having sex, he is touching her erogenous zones, and she realizes that she is not going to have an orgasm.

She pulls his hand up and says, "Just come inside me. I just want to feel you in me. I love to feel your pleasure." This is a code phrase for "You don't have to pleasure me. A quickie is fine because tonight my body is not in the mood for an orgasm."

10.	He is spending a lot of time on foreplay, and she really isn't in the mood for sex and just wants to feel close to him while he enjoys sex.	She can help guide him inside her, saying, "Let's have a quickie tonight."

Adding guilt-free quickies to your sex life provides an unexpected relief for both partners. Until a man experiences the freedom of never feeling the possibility of rejection, he won't know how it has been affecting him and holding back his passions. Using these new communication skills also frees a woman from having to perform or fake orgasm at those times when she discovers that she just isn't in the mood.

∽ **Why Men Stop Initiating Sex**

Each time a man initiates sex and is rejected, he's a little more hurt, his ego is a lit-

tle more bruised. After being burned and
spurned again and again, he hesitates to initiate sex and may even begin to lose touch
with his desire to have sex. He may begin
desiring other women who have not yet rejected him, or he may just lose interest. If he
is attracted to other women, he may mistakenly assume that he is no longer attracted to
his wife. If he just loses interest in sex, he
thinks it is because he is getting older.

〜

When a man feels repeatedly rejected in
sex, he begins to lose touch with his desire
to have sex. He may begin desiring other
women who have not yet rejected him,
or he may just lose interest.

〜

In the beginning of a relationship, couples
often have sex almost anytime they have the
opportunity. Then as the practicalities of
work and home come back into focus, natu-

rally there is less sex. Then with children, they have to schedule time or wait for an available moment.

When a man tries to initiate sex by saying, "Let's have sex," quite commonly a woman will unknowingly give any of the following rejecting messages:

"I can't right now. I need to make dinner."

"I can't right now. I have to return my calls."

"I can't. I have to go shopping."

"I don't have time."

"I can't. I already have too much to do."

"I'm not in the mood right now."

"This really isn't a good time."

"I have a headache."

141

"I can't think about sex right now."

"I have my period and I'm feeling crampy."

Each time this happens, a man will try to be understanding, but at a more primal emotional level, he finds it gets harder and harder to not feel rejected, and over time he may stop initiating sex. He may still want sex, but after being burned so often, he will hold back and wait for some clear sign from her that she is in the mood.

He may spend a lot of time trying to figure out when she seems open to sex, wondering, "Is this a good time to pursue?" Although he may not realize it consciously, every time he is in the mood and holds back from initiating sex, he ends up feeling more rejected.

❧ All Is Not As It Seems

Jake and Annie had been married for seven years. After about the first three years, they started having marital problems and sought help. They had started out passionately attracted to each other, and then over time the passion was gone. In counseling, Annie told Jake, "I miss having more sex with you. Is it something I did? Are you upset with me?"

He seemed surprised. "It seems to me like I always want sex and you don't. A lot of times when I want sex, I don't say anything because I know you are not in the mood."

She said, "How do you know if I am in the mood unless you ask?"

He said, "I can tell. I have been rejected enough."

She said, "That's really not fair. Sometimes if I am not in the mood, just by you mentioning that you want sex, I may discover that I am in the mood. Even if I don't feel in the mood right away, it helps me to move in that direction. I really appreciate when you initiate sex."

After Jake and Annie learned about guilt-free quickies, the passion came back into their relationship.

✒ Why Men Feel Rejected

When Annie and Jake talked about sexual rejection, she didn't readily understand why he would feel so rejected if she was not in the mood. She felt that because she truly loved having sex with him, he shouldn't feel rejected.

Intellectually, he agreed with that, but emotionally, it was very different. There are a variety of reasons that sexual rejection is one of the most sensitive and vulnerable areas for a man.

Biologically and hormonally, men are much more driven to be sexual than women are. Quite naturally, it is on their minds more of the time. Because a man is wanting it so much, he will feel rejected more of the time when he is not getting it.

✒

Because a man is wanting sex so much,
he will feel rejected more of the time
when he is not getting it.

✒

As we discussed before, it is primarily through sexual arousal that men begin to feel the most. A man's heart begins to open as he is turned on. When a man is aroused and about to initiate sex, he is most vulnerable. It is then that he can most deeply feel the pain of rejection. If he is already feeling hurt and rejected by his partner, arousal will make him feel that pain again. He may feel aroused and begin to feel angry and not even know why.

∽

If a man is already feeling hurt and rejected by his partner, arousal will make him feel that pain again. He may feel aroused and begin to feel angry and not even know why.

∽

When a man doesn't know how to avoid feeling rejected, it just increases his frustration and pain. As a result, he stops feeling attracted to his partner. If he doesn't consciously know how to solve this problem, to avoid feeling rejected, he unconsciously stops feeling turned on to his partner. This loss of attraction is not a choice but an automatic reaction.

In some cases, his sexual attraction is directed elsewhere to a fantasy woman who will not reject him or to a woman whom he doesn't care for. He is not risking a painful rejection if he doesn't care for the woman. This explains why a man can be turned on to a stranger but lose his attraction to the woman he loves most.

Women Love Sex

Women love sex, but before they can feel their desire for it, they have more requirements than men. A man doesn't readily understand this because throughout his life, he gets many messages that women don't like sex. To sustain passion and attraction in a relationship over the years, a man needs clear messages that she loves sex with him.

To sustain passion and attraction in a relationship over the years, a man needs clear messages that she loves sex with him.

As a general rule, men peak in their sexual interest when they are seventeen or eighteen years old. A woman reaches her prime when she is thirty-six to thirty-eight years old. It is similar to the pattern that men and women experience during sex. The man gets excited very quickly with little foreplay—except the opportunity to have sex—while a woman requires more time. Quite naturally, he feels that women don't like sex as much as he does.

His mother's attitude about sex may also influence him. If, as an adolescent, he was afraid of having his mother find out about his growing interest in sex and girls, he might have gotten the message that it is not OK to want sex. Later in life when he is with a woman that he cares about, these subconscious feelings can begin to emerge as little voices or faint feelings saying, "I can't be sexual around her or I will be rejected."

These past experiences may not directly cause a man to lose interest, but they certainly make him more sensitive to feeling rejected when she seems disinterested in sex. When she is not in the mood, subconsciously he begins to feel, "I knew it. She doesn't want to have sex."

One of the ways to counteract this tendency is for a woman to give the man repeated subtle messages that she likes sex. Her acceptance of occasional quickies is the strongest message of support she can give. Another powerfully positive message is to be very supportive whenever he initiates sex.

❦

**A *woman's* acceptance of occasional
quickies and a positive message
whenever her partner initiates sex
ensures lasting attraction and passion.**

❦

❦ How Men Unnecessarily Feel Rejected

Many times a woman is potentially in the mood for sex, but a man just doesn't realize it. He ends up feeling rejected when she might really want to have sex.

Sometimes a man will ask her any of the following questions:

"Would you like to have sex?"

"Do you want to have sex?"

"Are you in the mood for sex?"

To any of these requests, if she responds, "I'm not sure," or "I don't know," he will generally misunderstand and mistakenly hear rejection. He thinks she is politely saying no when she is really saying she doesn't know. This is hard for men to understand, because men are like the sun and not like the moon. When a man is asked if he wants sex, he has a definite response. The sun is either up or down. He generally knows for certain if he wants to have sex.

When a woman is unsure about wanting sex, it means that she needs a little time, attention, and talking to find out. With this new awareness, a man can easily overcome his tendency to immediately feel rejected and give up his pursuit.

∾ Is There a Part of You That Wants to Have Sex?

When a man's partner seems uncertain about having sex, instead of giving up, he should say, "Is there a part of you that wants to have sex with me?"

Almost always she will say yes. He may be surprised sometimes by how quickly she will respond by saying, "Sure, a part of me always wants to have sex with you." This will be music to his ears.

She may, however, then proceed to talk about all the reasons she doesn't want to have sex. She might say, "I don't know if we have enough time. I still have to do laundry and some errands." Or she might say, "I'm not sure how I am feeling. I have so much on my mind right now. I feel like I should devote time to finishing this project."

As she continues to talk, he should remind himself that she is not saying no. She just needs to talk, verbally sort things out, and then she can find her desire. Many times after sharing several reasons why she is not in the mood, she will then turn around and say, "Let's do it."

Without understanding how a woman is different, a man can easily feel turned off while she is talking about the reasons she doesn't know if she wants to have sex. But as long as he hears that a part of her wants to have sex, it is much easier for him to hear about the parts of her that don't want to have sex. Even if she finally discovers that she doesn't want sex, she can say, "We could have a quickie if you want and then some-time soon we can have (more leisurely) sex."

A woman can also use this insight. When a man wants to have sex and she is not sure, she can make it a lot easier for him to pa-tiently discover with her what she would like. Let's take an example:

He says, "Would you like to have sex?"

She says, "A part of me would love to have sex, but I'm not sure. I still have to buy groceries and then run some errands. I still haven't . . . etc."

Through first letting him know that a part of her wants to have sex, she makes it much easier for him to listen and accept the other reasons she may not be in the mood.

The Joy of "Quickies"

~

~ Is It Sex or Making Love?

Another way a man may get the message
that his partner doesn't like sex is if she never
uses the word "sex." Eric said, "I remember
in one relationship, my partner refused to call
sex, sex. She always wanted to call it 'making love.' When I called it 'sex,' she would
say no and become a little judgmental. She
didn't even want me to use the term. I could
understand that she liked the term 'making
love,' but I felt shamed by her. Certainly, my
heart and mind wanted to make love, but
my body wanted sex. After a while, I lost interest in sex with her. Eventually, we broke
up." This little semantics difference eventually created big problems.

When Eric went on to get involved with
Trish, he noticed that she often used the
term "making love" and not "sex." Having
already had some experience with this, he
decided to clear things up right from the beginning.

Eric told Trish that he really liked calling

sex, sex. He also told her that he understood that she liked the term "making love." They made a deal that she would be happy for him to use the word "sex" as long as when they had sex they would "make love," meaning that sex was always loving.

Occasionally, Trish would use the phrase "making love," which was OK with Eric, but it was very validating to him when she referred to it as "sex." Since they made their deal, when he uses the word "sex," he feels assured that she is completely OK with it.

Eric said, "If I had to say 'making love' instead of 'sex,' it would make me feel like I was somehow trying to fool her, or that in some way I had to hide that I wanted sex." Just this small difference in the way they referred to sex improved their sexual relationship.

The Joy of "Quickies"

~

~ Code Words for Sex

For some couples, the word "sex" has certain negative or painful connotations. If using the word "sex" is not comfortable, you can create secret code phrases. Even if the word "sex" is comfortable, you might like to do this anyway for fun.

One couple shared their code phrase with me in an interview. For them, the word "sailing" meant sex. Sometimes when the husband initiates sex, he says, "It's a sunny day. Would you like to go sailing?"

When she initiates sex, she says, "The weather looks really good today. Maybe we should go . . ." and he says, "Sailing?" They both smile and are ready to have a good time.

If "sailing" is your code word, then for long gourmet sex, you could say, "How about going for a long cruise?"

When he initiates sex and she is not in the mood, she could suggest a quickie by saying, "Let's use the speedboat instead." Be creative. See what fun code words you can share together.

∽ Sex and the Media

The media have a big effect on why men are so sensitive to rejection. A modern man is sensitive to feeling rejected sexually because each day he is bombarded with media advertisements featuring alluring sexual women whose bodies are saying, "Yes, I want you. I am ready for you. I long for you. I am yours. I want sex and more sex. Come and get me."

While this message is very exciting to a man, when he is caught up in this fantasy world, or when he is in the real world and thinking about his fantasy, he feels as if he is the only one not having hot and passionate sex. Even if he is in a relationship, he may feel that something is wrong when his sexual partner doesn't seem to be in the mood. The grass on the other side of the picture tube definitely seems greener.

A man does not realize that a woman really does want sex, but sometimes before she can feel her desires, she first needs his emotional support. When his partner doesn't want sex as much as he does, he begins to feel as if he has to jump through hoops to get it. He feels at a disadvantage because she doesn't want it as much.

She, however, does love sex but just needs to feel romanced and loved before her sexual needs can be just as strong as his. Sometimes awakening her sexual desires could be as simple as bringing home flowers for her or cleaning up the kitchen. (Don't laugh, men—in my seminars, women always clap loudly at this point!)

〜

A man does not realize that a woman really does want sex, but sometimes before she can feel her desires, she first needs his emotional support.

〜

The irony of modern times is that sex is everywhere in the media, and yet more and more I hear women complaining that their husbands are not interested in sex. The more sex men see in the media, the more rejected they begin to feel at home, and the more they lose attraction for their partners. A man loses attraction not because his partner doesn't measure up to the flawless female bodies he sees on TV or in magazines, but because he feels sexually rejected and frustrated.

It is vitally important for women to understand that it is not primarily the bodies men are attracted to but the message that these women are definitely open to having sex. To keep a man attracted to her, a woman does not need to compete with the fantasy women of the media and strive to create a perfect body. Instead, she needs to work toward communicating positive and nonrejecting messages about sex.

The Joy of "Quickies"

&

&

**To keep a man attracted to her, a woman
does not need to compete with the
fantasy women of the media and strive
to create a perfect body. Instead, she
needs to work toward communicating
positive and nonrejecting
messages about sex.**

&

& Why Men Feel at a Disadvantage

Without this understanding of the differences between men and women's sexual
needs, a man feels at a disadvantage. He
wants sex, but he feels that he has to convince the woman to want it as well.

He does not realize that she has a similar
disadvantage. Women hunger for intimacy
and good communication, and men don't
seem that interested. A woman can better

understand a man's sexual sensitivities by comparing them to her sensitivities about feelings, communication, and intimacy.

A *woman can better understand a man's sexual sensitivities by comparing them to her sensitivities about feelings, communication, and intimacy.*

It is a painful experience when a woman wants to talk but feels repeatedly rejected. Women can readily relate to this sensitivity. Without an understanding of the differences between men and women and the use of advanced skills to create better communication, his emotional withdrawing into his cave can be very painful for her. After a while, she doesn't even feel her needs to share and be open with him.

Just as a woman can apply new skills to

draw her partner out of the cave (see my book *Mars and Venus Together Forever*), a man can apply skills to open a woman up to sex. When we understand our differences, we realize that we are not trying to convince our partners to love us more or have sex with us on our terms, but rather we are supporting our partners by applying advanced skills. By successfully loving them, we enable them to give us the love we need.

Without these skills, after three or four years couples automatically lose the strong physical attraction they felt in the beginning. In the next chapter, we will explore why couples today are having less sex.

CHAPTER 7

Why Couples Are Having Less Sex

Couples today are having much less sex than the media suggest. Yes, a lot of hungry men and women are out there wanting sex, but once they are married, after a few years other things become more important and sex is overlooked.

The primary reason for this loss of interest is that men feel rejected and women don't feel romanced and understood in the relationship. A woman does not instinctively realize how sensitive a man is when she isn't in the mood for sex. A man does not instinctively realize how much a woman needs romance and good communication to open up and feel in the mood.

❧

The primary reason for loss of interest is that men feel rejected and women don't feel romanced and understood in the relationship.

❧

For men not to feel rejected, couples need to create free, positive, and easy communication about sex, particularly about initiating sex. When a man repeatedly gets the message and truly believes that his partner loves sex with him, his sexual desires can remain healthy and strong.

❧

When a man repeatedly gets the message and truly believes that his partner loves sex with him, his sexual desires can remain healthy and strong.

❧

❧

When a woman feels a man is skilled in sex and he supports her in the relationship, her sexual desire can remain fresh. Good communication and loving support in the relationship, however, are most important for a woman. For a man, a good relationship is certainly important, but many times what makes the big difference is his sexual success with her.

❧

When a woman feels a man is skilled in sex and he supports her in the relationship, her sexual desire can remain fresh.

❧

❧ Initiating Sex Versus Conversation

When a man is confident of his partner's positive feelings about sex, he will generally

167

keep initiating sex. If he feels that he is re-peatedly rejected or that he has to convince her to have sex, he will stop initiating. Even-tually, he will become sexually passive and less interested.

For a man to grow in passion, he needs to feel free to initiate sex. Just as a woman needs to feel that her partner will listen to her feelings in a positive way without reject-ing her, a man needs to feel he can initiate sex without being rejected.

When a man is not in the mood for conver-sation, he needs to say so gracefully. He can say, "I want to understand your feelings, but first I need some time alone, and then we can talk." When a man works to show he is interested in his partner's feelings and cares enough to come back and initiate conversa-tion, she feels loved.

In a similar way, when a woman is not in the mood for sex, but is careful to let him know that she loves sex with him, a man feels loved. When a woman is not in the mood, a man needs to hear that soon she will be back, ready and happy to have sex with him.

With this awareness, a woman automatically becomes more responsive to his sensitivity and is more motivated to find ways for him to feel free to initiate sex. Just as great communication opens a woman up to enjoy great sex, the possibility of great sex directly helps a man to be more loving in the relationship.

⬐

Just as great communication opens
a woman up to enjoy great sex,
the possibility of great sex directly
helps a man to be more loving
in the relationship.

⬐

⬐ When a Woman Wants More Sex

When a man doesn't initiate sex because he might get burned by rejection, he has to wait for her. When he feels he always has to wait for his partner to initiate sex, he eventually loses his desire and doesn't even know why. When this happens, the pendulum swings the other way, and he wants sex less than she does. Quite commonly, the woman begins to panic a bit.

She begins to miss sex and want it more. The more she wants it, however, the more he seems to lose his desire for it. Her desire for more becomes a message that he is not measuring up. Whatever desire he still has is quickly turned off.

Sex is a very delicate balance, and men are more vulnerable than women to an imbalance. If a man wants sex more than a woman does and can patiently persist in initiating sex respectfully, he will gradually win a woman over and sweep her off her feet, and automatically she will want to have sex.

When a woman consistently wants sex more than he does and expresses her unhappy feelings about it, a man can start to feel really turned off. He begins to feel as if he is obligated to have sex and has to perform for her.

Women already understand how performance pressure can numb their own arousal. With men, the effect of performance pressure is ten times greater.

A man cannot fake his arousal as a woman can. If he is not interested in sex, it is physically clear that he is not getting into it. A woman can easily hide her lack of arousal and pretend that everything is fine. A man cannot.

This increased sensitivity makes the pressure greater on a man. This greater pressure can immediately prevent him from getting aroused. If he feels he has to perform, nothing, and I mean nothing, happens down there.

❧

Because a man cannot fake his arousal as a woman can, he feels a greater pressure to perform.

❧

↬ What She Can Do When He's Not in the Mood

Many couples just give up at this point. The woman senses the embarrassment he feels and backs off. She doesn't know what to do. If she talks about it, he feels blamed, and if she makes sexual moves, he just feels tired or not in the mood.

Fortunately, there are solutions to this problem. Just as a man can share a quickie with his partner when she is not in the mood for sex, a woman can apply certain skills when her partner is not in the mood.

↬

Just as a man can share a quickie with his partner when she is not in the mood for sex, a woman can apply certain skills when her partner is not in the mood.

↬

At one point in their relationship, David and Sue found that she began to want sex a lot more than he did. Sue was frequently in the mood, and David happily responded when she initiated sex. For several weeks, everything worked great. They had sex several times a week and sometimes twice a day. Eventually, though, David began to wear out. This was a new experience for him. He had never felt a woman wanting it more than he did.

At first, he didn't know how to say no and would go ahead and have sex even if he didn't want to. This was not a good idea. Quite quickly, he began to feel pressure to perform. Sex was no longer fun. It was some kind of duty or obligation, and that just didn't feel good. To prevent feeling that way again, he decided he would have to say no.

It still wasn't clear to him how he could say no without rejecting Sue or hurting her feelings. When he came home from the office one evening, she cuddled up next to him on the couch while he was watching the news. After a few minutes, she started to gently stroke his thighs.

Trying not to be rude, he put his hand on hers to stop her movement and said, "I am so tired tonight. I really need to watch the news." Then, not wanting to sound too rejecting, he added without thinking, "Why don't you go upstairs and start, and then I'll join you later?"

David went back to watching TV and gradually forgot all about the exchange. He was tired and about ready to fall asleep when, forty-five minutes later, he heard a little voice from upstairs saying, "David, I'm ready."

It was like a miracle. Suddenly, from the waist down he was immediately awake. He said, "I'll be right up!"

When he got into bed, Sue was already prepared for an orgasm because she'd just spent the last forty-five minutes becoming more and more aroused, fantasizing about David making love to her while she caressed herself. It was no wonder that after about two minutes of penetration, she had an orgasm. A few seconds later, he had his. She was happy getting the sex she wanted, and it was a heavenly experience for David, even better than a quickie, because he didn't have to perform in any way and he still got to do the honors and give her an orgasm.

✑ Taking Responsibility for Our Own Pleasure

Instead of resenting that David was not in the mood, Sue just took responsibility for satisfying herself. This sense of responsibility is very healthy. Ideally, in all areas of a relationship, we should not make our partners responsible for our unhappiness, but particularly with sex it is very hard to satisfy our sexual needs without betraying our partners. This is why self-initiation is so important.

Sue's creativity freed her from feeling dependent on David when he couldn't be there for her the way she would have preferred. She made the best of the situation and got into bed and imagined him making love to her. Taking a long time to touch herself in a sensual way, she slowly built up her sexual tension so that when he joined her, she was already about to have an orgasm.

Afterward, he told her how much fun it was for him and that any time he was not in the mood, this was a great way to turn him on. This little conversation gave her permission to be much freer in her sexual expression and also ensured that she could have sex whenever she wanted it.

If a man is tired and not in the mood for sex, and she acts as if everything is fine, he really appreciates her easy acceptance. Otherwise, he might begin to feel the weight of performance pressure. If she is aroused and he's not in the mood, as he drifts off to sleep, she can just get into bed and begin to touch herself sensually.

After about twenty minutes, she can then turn on her side and gently but firmly rub up against his side. When he wakes up feeling her pressing on him, he can then move over to do the honors. In this way, they will both be happy. She never has to feel as if she can't get the sexual fulfillment she is looking for. This is why it's good for her to touch herself when he's around instead of just when she is alone.

If her partner travels a lot, she may occasionally want to give herself an orgasm while he is away. Knowing she can't wait may even turn him on more. Maybe he'll even start shortening his trips. I recommend that couples should let each other know when they are giving themselves orgasms so the partner can at least have the opportunity to join in.

Couples should let each other know when they are giving themselves orgasms so the partner can at least have the opportunity to join in.

✎ Getting Back to Sex

Many times when a couple stops having sex, it is hard to get back to it. The interruption could be due to a sickness, an argument, or a particularly stressful period of time, but after a couple loses the rhythm of sex, they may have a hard time getting back into the swing of things. It can be difficult to start again when you haven't had sex in a long while. If you use advanced skills, it won't be difficult to get back into the rhythm.

Jim had been out of work for several months and was feeling rather depressed. Julie, his wife of thirteen years, was frustrated not only that he was in his cave all the time, but also because they weren't having sex. Understanding his need for space, she worked hard at being very patient. Eventually, he got a new job and started feeling much better. Everything got better—except there was no sex.

I gave them a new approach to having sex again. I recommended that when she wanted sex, she say to him something along these lines: "I have been feeling really turned on today, and I can see that you're really tired. It's OK if you don't want to have sex, but I thought I would touch myself while thinking about you. As I get closer to having an orgasm, if you want to join in at any time, that will be fine with me. If you don't feel like it, that's OK too."

The next day, Julie called me and left a happy message on my machine. After many thanks, she said the new approach had worked like a charm. Jim also was very grateful. Sometimes it just takes one good experience, and a man is back in the saddle. There is no better aphrodisiac than sex itself. The easier it is to have sex, the more you want it.

❧ **The Indirect Approach**

Another secret for helping a man shift gears from not being interested in sex to feeling arousal is for a woman to be clear but indirect in her approach. Once you ask a man if he wants to have sex and he says no, it is much harder for him to shift and change his mind. As we have discussed, for women it is just the opposite. When you give her a chance to say no and talk about her feelings, she may start to become aroused and discover that she has changed her mind and does want sex.

Men tend to be very different. Once a man verbally says he doesn't want to have sex, to a certain extent it is written in stone. If she persists in her attempts to initiate sex, he feels controlled or pressured to perform.

Once a man verbally says he doesn't want to have sex, to a certain extent it is written in stone. If she persists in her attempts to initiate sex, he feels controlled or pressured to perform.

If, however, she can initiate sex in an indirect manner, he has time to silently overcome any resistance to having sex and possibly become aroused. To initiate sex in an indirect manner, a woman can develop various sexual signals. Even if he is in the mood and doesn't need time to gradually become aroused, he will still appreciate her signals, because they make it so much easier for him to initiate sex.

While these particular messages are very personal and may vary among women, here are some ways women can send sexual messages, particularly through what they wear to bed. The interpretations I give seem to be true for many, but, of course, every woman is ultimately unique and special.

BLACK LACE OR GARTERS

Wearing black lace or garters is one very clear signal that she wants sex. A revealing silky black outfit says she knows what she wants: not only does she want sex but she longs for it.

WHITE SILKY SATIN

When she wears white silky satin, she signals that she would like sensitive, gentle, and loving sex. It is as though she wants him to go slowly and be tenderly affectionate with her.

SILKY PINK OR LACE

When she wears silky pink or lace, she is ready to surrender to sex as a romantic expression of loving vulnerability and eventually wild abandon. She wants to feel his strength and surrender to his love. There is a deeper passion within her waiting to be drawn out that just needs to be ignited by his passionate longing and devotion to her.

SENSUOUS PERFUMES AND EXOTIC SMELLS

When she wears certain perfumes, she may want to be breathed in and savored in a sensuous way. For many men, a woman's sensuous perfumes and exotic smells can make sex much more lustful. He must be careful to control his passions and proceed slowly in sex, savoring each stage, occasionally pausing and repeating his previous actions before moving on to the next way of stimulating and pleasuring her.

BLACK BRA AND BLACK PANTIES

When she wears a black bra and black panties, she wants to be seductive, arousing, and perhaps more aggressive than usual. Although she begins strong, inside she wants him to dance with her but eventually end up in control of his passions as she lets go and surrenders to his love.

A SHORT AND LOOSE NIGHTGOWN WITH NO PANTIES

When she wears a short feminine cotton T-shirt and matching panties or a short and loose nightgown with no panties, it may mean she doesn't need a lot of foreplay tonight and she may or may not be in the mood for an orgasm. Maybe she just wants to feel close to him through intercourse.

GETTING INTO BED NAKED

When she gets into bed naked, after he initiates sex, she is open to discovering what kind of sex she is in the mood for, or she is simply open to whatever happens.

EARRINGS AND JEWELRY

When she wears earrings and other jewelry to bed, she feels beautiful and wants to be adored with lots of kisses. It may mean she wants very leisurely and sensual sex. He should remember to express verbally how beautiful she is many times.

OLD COTTON FLANNELS

When she wears old cotton flannels, clearly she is not in the mood! This is a particularly good time for cuddling. He can simply move closer and be physically affectionate and loving without becoming sexual.

Dressing for Sex

Through expressing her sexual feelings and moods in her dress, a woman greatly assists a man in feeling sexually wanted and welcomed. The messages listed above certainly are not exact for every woman, but they do provide a reference point for men to begin reading a woman's sexual signals. These examples may also assist women in becoming more conscious of the importance of dressing for sex in a way that is pleasing to him, but it must be pleasing and comfortable to her as well.

I personally became more aware of the messages my wife was sending me through the way she dressed for bed after a certain incident. After being affectionate for some time in bed, she got up, saying that she wanted to change. As she walked to the closet, I said, "Why bother changing? I am just going to take it off." She responded with a smile, "Yes, but I want you to take off the right outfit. This one really doesn't express how I feel today." From that point on, I became much more observant of what she wore and how it expressed her feelings and wishes in sex.

〜 **More Sexual Signals**

There are many more ways a woman can signal to a man that she is in the mood for sex without being too direct. Let's explore a few easy examples of how some women give their husbands a clear but indirect message when they are in the mood and open to sex.

Some of these messages may work for you, while others won't. Pick and choose as if you were in a store trying on outfits. They may even give you ideas to create your own messages as well.

RELAXING BATHS

Mary takes a long bath to let her partner, Bill, know she's in the mood. She brings in the portable CD player and plays the music that best fits her mood. Soft and gentle music means soft and gentle sex. Hard rock means she is in the mood for intense sex. Music with lots of drumbeats means she feels really sexy and wants it to last a long time.

CANDLES

Susan lights a candle by the bed or some incense when she is in the mood. Rachel lights candles for dinner when she is in the mood.

CHOCOLATES

When Sharon asks Tim to buy her a chocolate bar at the movies, he knows, "Tonight's the night." His wife tends to crave chocolate at those times when her body is desiring sexual release.

BUILDING FIRES

When she is in the mood, Carol lights a fire in the bedroom fireplace or asks her husband to build one. When he is building it, she sits and watches him and clearly lets him know how much she appreciates his taking the time.

STAYING UP

Usually when Grant arrives home late from a trip, Theresa has already gone to bed. Sometimes, however, she will stay up for him and be reading in bed when he gets home. If she clearly puts away her book when he walks into the room, he knows that she is in the mood.

MAKING HIS FAVORITE DINNER

Karen makes her husband's favorite salmon dinner with mashed potatoes when she is in the mood.

PISTACHIO NUTS

After a conversation during which Tom told Joyce that fresh pistachio nuts worked on him like an aphrodisiac, Joyce lets him know she is in the mood by bringing home fresh pistachio nuts from the market.

SPECIAL WINES

Margaret brings out a special wine that she and her husband really love. Sometimes she asks him to buy a bottle of it on his way home from work.

SNUGGLING

When Cheryl snuggles up to her husband while they are walking, he gets a clear message that she's in the mood.

THREE KISSES

When Maggie gives her husband a hello kiss, if she is in the mood, she will give him another two kisses. Three little kisses in a row, and he begins to feel the tingle that she is in the mood.

FOOT MASSAGE

Evelyn asks her husband for a foot massage when she is in the mood. Leslie signals that she is in the mood by offering to give her partner a foot massage. Either approach works.

⌒ *Putting Up the Flag*

My favorite example of sexual signals came from a movie I watched about a Mongolian family. When the wife was in the mood for sex, she would put out a flag. When her husband came home, he would see the flag and know that she was in the mood. He would then race to get his flag and hoop while she got on her horse and rode away. He would then get on his horse and chase after her, lasso her with his hoop, pull her off her horse, and wrestle with her. Then they would have sex. This little ritual definitely made for passionate sex. With her indirect but clearly stated permission, he would pursue her and take her. Although clearly in control, she could feel as if she were being pursued and eventually surrender herself in sexual passion and ecstasy.

❧ Positioning for Sex

Even where a woman gets undressed and ready for bed can be a very clear signal. If she undresses discreetly in front of her closet, she is generally not in the mood. But if she lays out her nightclothes on his side of the bed and undresses on his side of the bed so that he can clearly see her, it can be a definite message that she is in the mood.

When a woman positions herself to have sex by undressing in front of him, she may or may not get a response. If he is not in the mood, she is successfully preparing him to be aroused the next time.

If he is tired, instead of having to say, "I'm not in the mood" (which can be awkward for many men), he can just turn his head away into his pillow and let out a sigh, saying, "Ahhh, I am so glad to get into bed. I am so tired." This is a clear message that he is not in the mood.

She is spared from directly being rejected, and he is spared from having to say he doesn't want to have sex. The last thing he wants is for her to interrogate him with a series of questions expressing her concern.

When Questions Are a Turnoff

Asking a man a series of questions about why he is not in the mood is not only an immediate turnoff, but can prevent him from being in the mood in the future. These are some questions not to ask if he doesn't respond to your sexually inviting signals.

"What's wrong?"

"Don't you want to have sex with me anymore?

"You used to always want sex."

"Do you think I am getting fat?"

"Are you still attracted to me?"

"Aren't you turned on to me?"

"Do you still love me?"

"Maybe we should talk about it."

"Maybe we should get some help."

"Are we ever going to have sex again?"

"You were looking at other women tonight. Don't you want to be with me anymore?"

"Would you rather be with someone else?"

"Did I do something to turn you off?"

194

Why Couples Are Having Less Sex

~

"Why don't you want to have sex?"

"What's the matter, is something wrong?"

Certainly there may be appropriate times she can ask these questions, but they are definitely not recommended when she has just undressed in front of him and he is tired and turning away from her. Instead, she should respond at this most sensitive moment as if everything is fine and OK. This is not the time for her to seek his reassurance.

By being neutral and indirect, she can more successfully maintain the nondemanding message that she is welcoming him if he happens to be in the mood.

If he is not in the mood, she can go to bed knowing that they will have sex soon. If, however, she is really in the mood, she can just take matters into her own hands. It is very important that a man support a woman's need to do so, in order that she doesn't ever feel deprived of having an orgasm if her body happens to be wanting one when he is not in the mood.

This mutual understanding works like a charm. If he knows he is welcome to join in at any time or simply go to sleep, he will tend to wait till she is almost about to have her orgasm and then join in. This method works because there is no pressure on him.

After hearing about this approach, a man may decide to reassure his partner that it's fine with him if she wakes him up and includes him right before she is about to have her orgasm.

〜 **When Men Stop Initiating Sex**

One of the major reasons a couple stops having sex is that a man stops initiating sex or a woman initiates sex too much. When a woman does all the initiating, not only does she gradually become frustrated, but after a while a man will begin to lose interest in sex with her.

Why Couples Are Having Less Sex

～

Women generally do not understand that if they pursue a man more than he pursues her, the man will eventually become more passive. A little pursuing energy is fine to let him know when it is a good time for him to pursue her, but when she does it all, he loses interest and doesn't even know why.

When a woman feels too responsible for initiating sex, a man slowly begins to feel less motivated. When she expresses her masculine pursuing side, he moves too far to his feminine receptive side. This imbalance slowly erodes the passion in a marriage.

Quite commonly, he doesn't even know what happened to his passionate feelings for his partner, and he may even mistakenly assume that he simply is no longer attracted to her. When a women initiates sex in an indirect manner, as I have pointed out, she ensures that her partner can find his masculine side that desires her and seeks to pursue her.

~

**When a woman initiates sex in an
indirect manner, she ensures that her
partner can find his masculine side that
desires her and seeks to pursue her.**

~

Most men have no idea that too much assertiveness and sexual aggression on her
part can eventually turn him off. Some men
like a woman's assertiveness very much at
first but then have no idea why they are no
longer attracted to her or suddenly find
other women more attractive. In the beginning, a sexually assertive woman may feel
great for him because he feels relieved that
he doesn't have to risk rejection, but over
time, his passion will lessen.

Women commonly complain that they
don't want to always initiate sex. My sug-
gestion is that instead of initiating sex, a
woman can focus on giving a man the message that it is safe for him to initiate sex.

〜

〜

Instead of initiating sex, a woman can focus on giving a man the message that it is safe for him to initiate sex.

〜

There is no problem with a woman initiating sex *some* of the time. It becomes a problem when she initiates sex *more* of the time. Gradually, he will initiate sex less and lose interest.

〜 When Women Aren't Interested in Sex

Men feel discouraged when they feel that their wives don't seem to make sex as important as they do. Without consistent clear messages from her that she enjoys sex, he may lose his attraction to her. Suddenly, women he doesn't know, who haven't yet rejected him, become more attractive.

Historically, men have been much more sexually active outside a marriage than women. Without good communication and romantic skills, couples lose a great degree of their sexual interest in each other. While women might have sought fulfillment in their fantasies, men acted out their frustrated feelings and fantasies through having affairs.

In the past, women could more easily give up the need for sex in favor of the routine requirements of creating a home and family. The survival of the family was more important than the fulfillment of sexual passions. Sexual fulfillment was a luxury women couldn't afford. Men coped with the lessening of women's sexual interest by discreetly finding sex elsewhere.

Unfortunately, as soon as a man directs his energies elsewhere, it is much harder for his partner to feel emotionally fulfilled enough to direct her sexual passions toward him. As a result, the family unit was preserved, but romance was lost.

❧

The major reason men would resort to affairs is that they did not understand that they had the power to reawaken their partner's sexuality.

❧

The major reason men would resort to affairs is that they did not understand that they had the power to reawaken their partner's sexuality. They did not have the skills that we can now apply. With a deeper understanding of the opposite sex, we can now rekindle the flame of passion even when it has blown out. In the next chapter, we will explore how to rekindle the passion in a relationship.

CHAPTER 8

How to Rekindle the Passion

Many times a couple may feel sexually attracted to each other during the day when they're apart, but when they get home, they lose the feeling. For example, a husband at work may miss his wife and feel aroused, but when he gets home, he loses the attraction. A woman may feel as if she also wants more romance, but when she gets home, the feeling is gone.

This occurrence may be due to a variety of reasons. It could simply be that the domestic responsibilities of managing the home or children overshadow the romantic feelings. Too much routine can lessen the passion.

It may also be that some little unresolved feelings linger after an uncomfortable conversation or argument. To a great extent, the issue may have been resolved, but it wasn't resolved in an ideal way. The disagreement is easily forgotten outside the home, but when the couple is at home, it comes back in a vague way, and suddenly the attraction is gone. When you rekindle the passion in your relationship, the love shared while having sex can wash away these little stains and smooth out rough edges.

Although as a general rule of thumb the relationship comes first before sex can be enjoyed, sometimes having loving sex can dramatically improve the relationship. A woman's openness to having sex can open up a man's love for her. Sometimes even if she is feeling cold, having sex with him and feeling his love for her in sex can open her up again.

∽

*Although as a general rule of thumb
the relationship comes first before sex
can be enjoyed, sometimes having
loving sex can dramatically
improve the relationship.*

∽

Perhaps the partners are simply out of the habit of having sex regularly. Outside the home, they are free to feel their sexual desires, but in the home, the old routine of not having sex takes over. Once sex gets put on a back burner, it becomes harder to bring back without advanced relationship skills. With a greater awareness of what skills are needed, even when the passion is gone, it is often very easy to rekindle.

∽ Romantic Getaways

One of the simplest and most powerful ways to rekindle passion is to get out of the house on a romantic getaway. Spend the night at a hotel. Enjoy a change of scenery. Get away from the routine and familiar. Temporarily leave all domestic responsibilities behind. The more beautiful the new environment is, the better.

Try to get away at least one night once a month. If you can't visit a vacation spot or a neighboring town, go to a local hotel. Sometimes just getting into a different bed can do the trick.

Women particularly often need a change of environment to be aroused. This change frees the woman from feeling responsible for the family and the home. When the environment is beautiful, it awakens her to her inner beauty.

〜

〜

Women particularly often need a change of environment to be aroused.

〜

〜 When to Get Away

Quite commonly, a man will make the mistake of waiting until his partner gives clear messages that she wants sex before he plans a little getaway. This is a big mistake. The getaway helps her to get in the mood. If he waits for her to feel sexy before planning a getaway, then he may just wait and wait, and things will just get worse.

If, for a long time, a woman has not been able to get away and feel free to be romantic and sexual, her mood may become increasing asexual. To reignite the passion and to feel like a beautiful and loved woman, she needs to get away from the daily responsibilities and routine. Just by scheduling the getaway, it may begin to bring back her romantic feelings.

A man needs to remember that sometimes before a woman can feel romantic, she needs to talk. If it is a long drive to the vacation spot, she can talk the whole way. Women particularly need to talk to let go of stress and leave it behind.

After this kind of long drive in which she can unwind, she's likely to arrive at your vacation spot and your new bedroom in a great mood. Suddenly, a whole new feeling emerges that could not have come up at home. She might want sex right away, or she might want to go for a walk or enjoy eating out. But once she starts feeling taken care of, she can stop feeling as if she has to take care of others. In this way, her inner passions are awakened.

Another way to help her relax is to take her shopping, if that is something she enjoys. Although this can be very tiring for men, most women's stores now have chairs for a man to sit in while she tries on outfits.

～

Just the act of exploring a store and gently reflecting on what she likes and what she wants helps her to shift from being concerned about others to feeling her own needs. Even if she doesn't buy anything she can still be happy.

A woman directly benefits from the process of exploring what she wants. This helps her understand her likes, wishes, and desires, and directly prepares her for experiencing passion and desire. A little shopping can greatly add to the joys of getting away.

If she is enjoying herself and appreciating everything, a man will probably be easily aroused as well. When she enjoys the new environment, an emotional part of him takes credit for her happiness. This feeling of success can awaken his feelings of arousal. Leaving their problems behind in this way, they can enjoy each other more fully.

While spontaneous getaways can rekindle the romantic spirit, sometimes we are just too busy or responsible to others to get away easily. When getaways are scheduled, a

woman can stay more in touch with her sexual desires. That part of her can look forward with certainty to being fulfilled.

Writing a Romantic Letter

Another secret for bringing back sexual
feelings is to write a romantic letter to your
partner. If you find that when you are away
from your partner, you are interested in sex,
but when you are home you are not turned
on, practice writing down your sexual feelings when they arise. As I mentioned, domestic stresses can easily overshadow and
lessen sexual feelings. The sexual feelings
may be inside us, but they need a little extra
help to come out in the home.

When you are away from your partner,
feel your aroused mood and imagine a romantic scene acting out those sexual feelings with your partner. In a letter to your
partner, describe what you want to do and

then describe the scene and your feelings as if it is really happening.

∽ When You Are Not a Writer

Of course, many people are not writers, and expressing these delicate sentiments may be difficult. That does not mean the feelings don't exist; it just means that you are not gifted in expressing them in words. Women particularly love to hear these emotions in words. That is one reason women spend billions of dollars buying romance novels.

A man who has difficulty verbalizing his passion might want to buy a greeting card that poetically expresses how he feels. It is perfectly normal to have loving feelings and not know how to articulate them and do justice to them. Picking the right card to express your feelings is just as good as writing the words yourself.

Picking the right card to express your feelings is just as good as writing the words yourself.

This same principle holds true with romantic letters. Feel free to borrow many of the words and expressions from romance novels. It is more important to capture your feelings and express them in words than to be original.

After you have written your letter, tell your partner you have a special letter to share. Schedule some special time—at least forty-five minutes without any interruptions—so that you can read the letter or your partner can read it (either aloud or silently). Quite automatically, those feelings will come back as the letter is read, and you can then enjoy great sex again.

This technique has helped me and my wife many times to rekindle our sexual feelings for each other. I did not realize how important it was to Bonnie until once she shared with me that she kept these letters in a very special spot, and when she didn't feel loved by me, she would bring them out and read them again.

Romantic letters are not only good for getting sex going but can also help your partner understand how you feel when you are having sex. Without these letters, Bonnie would have never known so definitely the depth of my passion for her during great sex.

~ In the Middle of the Night

A combination of great sex and the quickie is doing it in the middle of the night. It is a wonderful feeling for a man to have his wife wake him up in the middle of the night by pressing herself against him.

A woman who is feeling in the mood might want to take twenty to thirty minutes touching herself until she is almost about to have an orgasm, then move over to his side

of the bed. He'll find this a particularly wonderful way to wake up.

Since he only needs a few minutes to be
aroused and she has taken time to stimulate
herself, they both get to have pleasure. If a
man wants sex with his partner in the middle of the night, however, it is not the same,
because she doesn't wake up ready to go in
a few minutes.

It is, however, an incredibly liberating experience for him to feel free sometimes to
reach over and have sex with her. This kind
of freedom is wonderful, but certain conditions need to be met first. There must be
openness to regular sex and regular loving
communication before you try this technique.

He needs to ask her at another time if she
is open to being awakened. She may not
want to be awakened unless she is on vacation and is very rested or can sleep late.

Even with her consent, when a man
wakes up his partner, he must be less aggressive about it than she would be in wak-
ing him up. If he is turned-on in the night,
he can gently begin to move over to his wife,

slowly touching her, holding her and rubbing against her. If she opens herself to him, it is OK, but she must also feel that it is perfectly OK for her to say, "Not tonight."

If a man can hear, "Not tonight" without feeling rejected, it is safe for her to say it. If she doesn't feel safe to say no to sex, she automatically loses her ability to really say yes to sex. There is no greater way to lessen sexual attraction than to have sex when you don't want to.

〜

If a woman doesn't feel safe to say no to sex, she automatically loses her ability to really say yes to sex.

〜

Through respecting each other's unique sexual needs, both partners can give and receive the support they need. In the next chapter, we will explore an approach to sex that ensures that both partners are always satisfied.

CHAPTER 9

Polarity Sex

Another secret for great sex and keeping the passion alive is understanding and working with our different sexual polarities. Just as the negative pole of a magnet strongly attracts the positive pole of another magnet, by expressing our opposite sexual polarities, we can increase attraction, desire, and pleasure.

There are two sexual polarities, giving pleasure and receiving pleasure. When one partner is giving and the other partner is receiving, the sexual pleasure can easily build. In polarity sex, partners take turns consciously using these polarities to increase desire and pleasure. One partner gives while the other receives. Then, later on, they switch, and the giver stops giving and just receives.

Polarity sex has two stages. In the first stage, the man takes and the woman gives. Then, in the second stage, he attends to her needs while she relaxes and focuses on receiving.

While practicing the first stage of polarity sex, the man starts out receiving. He is not primarily concerned with spending a lot of time providing her with pleasure. Certainly, he wants her to enjoy it, but he is really focused on his own pleasure. Likewise, she is not expecting herself to get turned on right away and keep up with him.

In the second stage, it is her turn to receive while he focuses on giving. She has done all her giving, and now she can just receive. In this way, both people eventually get everything they want.

∾ **Developing Polarity Sex**

I first developed the idea of polarity sex because I know a man doesn't *always* want to take a long time giving his sexual partner the foreplay she may need to have an orgasm. It is not that he doesn't care about her pleasure, just that his body wants to get on with it. This difference in time needed for foreplay sometimes creates a big problem.

Focusing on himself without giving her the foreplay she needs only builds resentment on her part. Yet waiting for her might create frustration for him. If he just goes for it, after his orgasm his energy will be spent, and his partner will be left with very little of what she needs. After a while, he'll stop wanting sex because he doesn't want to take the time for foreplay. Sometimes a man is just tired at the end of the day and doesn't have the patience. The thought of having to do all that foreplay can be a turnoff.

In a similar way, many times a woman doesn't want to have sex because she doesn't want her partner to be frustrated as he tries to quickly bring her to orgasm. For the thought of sex to be a welcome idea, a woman needs to feel that she doesn't have to get turned on right way. She doesn't always know how long it will take or if it will even happen that time.

For the thought of sex to be a welcome idea, a woman needs to feel that she doesn't have to get turned on right way. Polarity sex is the solution to this problem.

Polarity sex is the solution to this problem, and as we will see, it has many other advantages as well. Instead of feeling frustrated that he has to wait for his partner's sexual pleasure to build up, a man can at first just go for it and do whatever turns him on. Then, before he is about to have an orgasm, he should stop and start over to give her all the foreplay she needs to build up her desire. Then, after giving her an orgasm, he can easily have his.

∽ Practicing Polarity Sex

Polarity sex often starts with the man feeling aroused and aggressive about releasing his sexual tension, and the woman simply enjoying his arousal. He may hold his lover, kiss her, touch her, undress her, and become increasingly excited by her. She might just lie there enjoying being so desirable to him, or she might begin to touch him in ways that excite him.

She does not feel that she has to match his level of excitement. Instead, she just supports him in being excited. She can get involved in stimulating him, particularly by touching, holding, and stroking him. All this is to build up the man's sexual excitement. In a very clear way, he is receiving or taking pleasure, and she is giving it to him.

After about five minutes, as his excitement begins to peak and he can tell that orgasm is approaching, he signals for her to stop stimulating him. He might signal that he is getting close to an orgasm by making a strong sound like "ooohhh" or taking a deep breath, relaxing on the exhale and gently pulling away from her touch to change positions.

To signal that he is ready to switch the polarity, he can simply move her hands back and place them over her shoulders. In addition, he may also gently switch sides of the bed.

Each of these signals says clearly to her that now he is ready to give back all the pleasure she has given him. She can relax and begin to focus on her body and her pleasure as he slowly begins to arouse her body. Although he might only need two or three minutes of stimulation, he needs to remind himself that she needs twenty to thirty minutes.

～

**Although a man might only need
two or three minutes of stimulation
to approach orgasm, he needs to
remind himself that a woman needs
twenty to thirty minutes.**

～

～ Shifting the Polarity

In the beginning, it may be hard for him to
stop and shift polarities by moving to stage
two. He might get too excited. This particularly happens when she gives him oral sex
or they are having intercourse in stage one.
By understanding her need for him to be
aroused when she has her orgasm, he can
find the control he needs.

❧

**By understanding her need for him to be
aroused when she has her orgasm, he
can find the control he needs.**

❧

Women and men are biologically wired to
have a different experience after orgasm.
After a woman has an orgasm, she is still
aroused and can enjoy intercourse even
more. After her orgasm, her pleasure hormones* stay at a very high level. After his orgasm, a man generally loses his arousal
quickly. When he is done, he is done. His
pleasure hormones to a great extent dissi-
pate and disappear.

If he has an orgasm first, his energy is not
there for her when she is ready to have hers.
If she has her orgasm first, not only is she
still sexually aroused, but she can enjoy his
orgasm more.

---

*Endorphins, catecholamine, and neurotransmitters.

∿ Timing Orgasms: Ladies First

Many times couples will try to schedule their orgasms to occur at the same time. This kind of timing can actually make sex less fulfilling. It is very distracting for a woman to be concerned about when she is going to have an orgasm. It is best for her to feel free to discover it when it comes without having to adjust herself and try to control it. After she's had her orgasm, he can then have his right away or wait a little.

When a man and woman climax together, both individuals are so absorbed with their intense pleasure that in a way the partner is momentarily gone, and the intimacy suddenly disappears.

∿

When a man and woman come to orgasm together, sometimes it can be less fulfilling.

∿

One minute a woman is enjoying the full extent of his attention, and the next minute it is gone. Likewise, when a man feels the pleasure of his own orgasm, he misses experiencing the full extent of her pleasure. Until his orgasm suddenly comes, he fully experiences her increasing pleasure. When his orgasm comes, he is too caught up in the intensity of his own experience of pleasure to feel the full development and expression of her pleasure and her love for him.

If he times it so that she can have an orgasm first, because he remains in control, he helps her to go further out of control. When she has her orgasm, he can fully be there with her to completely enjoy her pleasure. Then, once she has had her orgasm, she is free to fully experience his. It is like having two orgasms instead of just one. Both partners fully experience her orgasm, and then both partners fully experience his.

If he has an orgasm first, to fully experience his pleasure, she is distracted from her own gradual buildup and then, if she does eventually have an orgasm, he is definitely unable to fully feel her orgasm because he is no longer completely aroused. Through following the general guidelines of polarity sex, a woman is assured each time that she will at least have the opportunity to have an orgasm. Sometimes she may discover that she is not going to have one, but because he has spent the time without burdening her with expectations, she is quite fulfilled.

⌒

Through following the general guidelines of polarity sex, a woman is assured each time that she will at least have the opportunity to have an orgasm.

⌒

⌒ **Bonus Benefits of Polarity Sex**

A bonus benefit of polarity sex is that after a man has taken his pleasure in phase one, when it is her turn a woman naturally feels more entitled to receive her pleasure. Without this extra feeling of entitlement, some women find it difficult to achieve orgasm.

Many times, when a women is particularly good at giving to others, she has a difficult time receiving. In sex, she may be so busy thinking about her partner's need or so concerned for him that she doesn't give herself permission to focus on her own needs. This tendency can be completely unconscious. Once when I was describing this point in one of my seminars, a woman suddenly became very animated and exclaimed, "I can't believe it. . . . That's it." Everyone could tell she had had an "ah ha" experience and wondered what it was.

I stopped and asked her what had happened. This is her story:

> I just realized why I had my only orgasm. I am forty-two years old, and I have never had an orgasm with a partner except once. I never could understand why, and now I know. About six years ago, my partner

wanted to have sex with me. However, I was feeling resentful. I felt I had given much more in our relationship. After he persisted, I decided to have sex but planned to only receive and enjoy being touched.

When we had sex, he did everything for me, but for the first time in my life, I did nothing for my sexual partner. I told myself this was for me and really had the time of my life. Now I understand why I had an orgasm—because I wasn't focusing on giving him pleasure, I could focus on myself, and it worked. Even though I did nothing to please him, he also was quite happy as well.

As this example points out, when a woman can fully receive, she can really enjoy sex. Polarity sex helps her to receive because after she clearly gives to him she can then shift to receiving. By having the mutual understanding of polarity sex and a clear signal that phase two has begun, a woman can more fully relax and enjoy the gradual buildup of her sexual fulfillment.

❧ When a Man Is in Control

When a man is in control of his pleasure so that it doesn't become so great that he has an orgasm before she does, a woman can enjoy sex even more. She does not have to be concerned with having to hurry up so she can achieve orgasm before he is done.

The more she knows he is in control and not going to climax before she does, the more she can fully relax and let go. This is another advantage of polarity sex. In phase one, he gets his pleasure but doesn't have an orgasm. Then, in phase two, she knows the rest of the time is for her. She can relax, knowing that he will be there for her.

❧

***The more she knows he is in control and
not going to come before she does, the
more she can fully relax and let go.***

❧

Sometimes in sex a man feels a strong urge to have an orgasm before a woman does. At these times, he must not allow her to stimulate his penis. He needs to pull back from stimulation and calm down. This calming down is done in two ways.

First, he needs to pull away from being stimulated before it is too late. Then he can begin to increase stimulation of her. Increasing her pleasure to the level of his pleasure will actually allow him to regain control.

Sometimes a woman really loves it if he gives her an orgasm before intercourse. This means that he gets excited in phase one, then in phase two he brings her to orgasm, and then they have intercourse, and he can have his orgasm. When he enters her after her orgasm, he is very, very welcome.

❦ After a Woman's Orgasm

After a woman has had her orgasm, she can actually enjoy his penetration the most because she is not only more open to being stimulated, but she can enjoy his pleasure more. She has had her release, and now she can focus on receiving and loving him. For her at this point, it is a different kind of stimulation. Before orgasm, she experiences a mounting pleasure, but after orgasm, it is as if she has climbed the mountain and is dancing on top of the world with her partner.

At this stage he is free to move in and out of her without any performance pressure. He could take one minute or ten, and she will be completely happy. To a woman, it doesn't matter how long a man lasts if he first satisfies her. Sometimes men misunderstand a woman's need and mistakenly assume longer is better. Generally speaking, intercourse longer than thirty minutes will make a woman very sore.

Men feel a great deal of pressure to last a long time so that she will get the stimulation she needs. By practicing polarity sex, she is always assured that she will get the time she needs before he comes.

〰

**To a woman, it doesn't matter how long
a man lasts if he first satisfies her.**

〰

〰 **Increasing a Woman's Pleasure**

A man tends to think in a very goal-oriented
way. He wants to provide increased pleasure
for a woman in the most efficient way possible. Once she is getting close to orgasm, he
continues stimulating her to push her over
the edge and achieve the goal. The secret of
giving her more pleasure is to bring her
close to orgasm and then pull back, slow
down, lessen stimulation, and then start
over.

To most effectively build a woman's pleasure, a man should bring her to the point of
orgasm and then let her energy settle down,
then bring her back up, and then let her settle down. If he brings her to the verge of or-

gasm two or three times and then finally gives her an orgasm, it will be much bigger and more fulfilling.

Each time she gets closer, her longing and desire for orgasm increases. Her body also gets a chance to fully prepare for the orgasm. By extending foreplay in this way, not only does she experience a bigger orgasm, but his orgasm is much more intense as well.

In polarity sex, a man should first build his energy toward his orgasm. Then when he pauses and focuses on her, his energy will relax. Later on, when it is his turn to have an orgasm, his pleasure will be much greater because he has waited.

One way a woman can signal to a man that she is about to have an orgasm is to use the code word, "Please." The word has a double meaning: "Please stop or I will have an orgasm," and "You are pleasing me so much." When he gets the signal, he can choose to continue and give her an orgasm or lessen direct stimulation for thirty seconds to a few minutes before he brings her up again.

When he pauses, it is not as if everything has to stop. He can continue touching her all over her body in a very erotic way without directly touching her between the legs. This gives her a chance to let her energy settle down a bit before he takes it even higher.

✎ Expanding Our Pleasure Potential

Each time we allow the energy to settle down before building it up, we are expanding the body's ability to enjoy pleasure. I once did an experiment that is analogous to this point.

A friend of mine had a pain clinic. To lessen chronic pain, the doctor would first place a needle in the patient's body at a certain key point. Then a current of electricity would be sent into the patient's body through the needle. Over a one-hour period, the current flow would be dramatically increased. It was amazing how much more electric current the body could accept if the flow was slowly increased. Although I was not experiencing chronic pain, I wanted to see what this treatment felt like.

They put the needle in my arm, then slowly turned up the electricity until I felt a burning pain. At that point, I signaled that it was too much, and they reduced it a little and then left it at that more comfortable level.

After ten minutes, a nurse came and turned a knob that immediately doubled the intensity. I could feel a difference, but it didn't burn at all.

Because the electricity flow was first at my maximum tolerance, then was decreased a little and kept at that point for ten minutes, my body had time to adjust and open up to receive more current. In just ten minutes, I could receive twice as much electric current. I was amazed.

After another ten minutes, the nurse came back and again increased the flow by the original amount. After just twenty minutes, I was easily able to accept three times the original amount.

Every ten minutes for an hour, the flow was increased. After an hour, I could receive without shock or pain six times the original amount. By slowly adapting to the current, my body could take six times more current. This was a typical response.

The next day, I returned to the pain clinic and started with the same amount that I had begun with the day before. Then I decided to turn the current up further anyway and doubled the amount right away instead of waiting ten minutes. I ended up shocking and burning myself. I was able to clearly experience the body's ability to adapt and receive more current if given the time.

In a similar way in sex, if we take the time to build up the energy and then get used to it and then build again, the ability to experience pleasure dramatically increases. By building up the energy and then pausing, we are actually expanding our container of pleasure so that we can experience greater enjoyment and have bigger and more fulfilling orgasms.

❧

By building up the energy and then pausing, we are actually expanding our container of pleasure so that we can experience greater enjoyment and have bigger and more fulfilling orgasms.

❧

When you take the time to build up pleasure again and again, you often have a full body orgasm. If you get excited and go straight for a quick orgasm, it is generally more concentrated in the genital area and not nearly as grand.

❧ Healthy Home-Cooked Sex and Gourmet Sex

Unless they are having a quickie, a man should bring his partner up at least two or three times before giving her an orgasm.

Polarity Sex

∿

This is a dietary staple of great sex and takes about thirty minutes.

Healthy home-cooked sex takes about thirty minutes. Five minutes for him, twenty minutes for her to build to orgasm, and then, after he reaches orgasm, five minutes to enjoy the afterglow of lying together in love.

It is good to know clearly that sex can be mutually satisfying for both partners in a relatively short period of time. If sex takes hours and hours, the passion will eventually die out. We begin to associate sex with a lot of time, and in our busy schedules, it is too difficult to find that much time. But even in a busy schedule, a half hour is easy to schedule at least once or twice a week.

In addition to home-cooked sex, it is important to create a window of privacy when you have at least two hours to enjoy gourmet sex. During gourmet sex, you can take turns bringing each other up to the point of orgasm. For example, she might start by bringing him up, then he takes her up a few times, then she can take him up again. Going back and forth, they can extend the foreplay until, eventually, she can't hold back anymore.

For a man, not only is gourmet sex wonderful, but it trains him to control his sexual energy. Not only is it more pleasurable, but it also gives him the new experience of slowing down and being more in the moment.

After you go up several times, the urgency for climax lessens, and you can begin to savor every moment, every taste, every smell, every breath, every little sound, every sensation. In addition, you can more fully experience the flow or current of love to and from your partner.

During gourmet sex, however, a couple will spend more time in phase one. The man might come close to climax several times. Then they will shift to phase two, and she will come close to orgasm again and again. Then they might move back into phase one. Eventually, as their bodies gradually open up to receive more sexual electricity, they can enjoy giving and receiving at the same time. Although you don't have to follow the guidelines of polarity sex rigidly, do make sure that the woman has her orgasm first.

❧ Quickie Sex

Quickie sex takes about three to five minutes. It is basically just phase one of polarity sex and is all for his pleasure. A woman is generally open to occasional quickie sex when she feels emotionally supported in the relationship and knows that at other times she will experience regular healthy home-cooked sex and occasional gourmet sex.

❧

A woman is generally open to occasional quickie sex when she feels emotionally supported in the relationship and knows that at other times she will experience regular healthy home-cooked sex and occasional gourmet sex.

❧

Regular quickie sex may appeal only to him, but it has extra benefits for her as well. Although she doesn't experience the physical stimulation of longer sex, emotionally it can be very fulfilling for a woman for a variety of reasons.

Since I began teaching how and why to incorporate quickies into a couple's sex life, not only men have thanked me but women as well. These are some examples of what women have told me:

"Now when we are having sex and I discover I am not in the mood, I don't have to fake it, I can just say, 'Let's have a quickie.' He doesn't get bummed out, and I don't have to explain that there is nothing wrong."

"It's great because sometimes I just want to be close and cuddle, but I also want him to be satisfied as well. I get to be close, but I don't have to try and get into it."

"Finally he understands that sometimes I just like to have intercourse and I don't care about having an orgasm."

"Quickies are great. I don't have to worry about how turned on I have to get. Sometimes we start out in a quickie and I start getting really turned on. I just tell him I want him to touch me, and he is very happy to shift gears and give me an orgasm. I would have never known I was in the mood if we hadn't started out in a quickie."

"I used to tell him that I didn't have to have an orgasm, but I did like having sex if he was in the mood. He used to get upset, like something was wrong. Then when he heard your tapes on sex, everything changed. Somehow, because someone else told him, he could really hear. Now, without feeling pressured to perform each time, I have started enjoying sex much more, and now I feel like having an orgasm much more often."

"Sometimes I don't want sex to be this long process. I want to get it over with. Instead of having to fake an orgasm to finish up, I can just tell him, 'Let's have a quickie,' and in a few minutes we are done."

"Sometimes when we go out, there are a lot of younger women around. Even if I am not in the mood for sex, I do enjoy feeling that I still turn my partner on. I will initiate sex at those times with some clear signals. Then as we start, I let him know he doesn't need to stimulate me much. It feels good to feel my man wanting and desiring me."

These kinds of comments add a new awareness to the importance of quickies.

∽ **How Many Orgasms Are Enough?**

Many books today talk about achieving more and more orgasms. Although these books are certainly helping some couples, many women just feel more pressure to perform. With our busy schedules, it is enough to think about having one orgasm. Now in the nineties, women are expected to have many.

Many women are completely satisfied with one orgasm. Sometimes more of something is not better. When a woman is satisfied with one orgasm, the man giving her that one orgasm is also very satisfied. In a way, he can feel, "I did that. I completely satisfied her."

Some women go on and on, one orgasm after another. Although a man might find this very exciting, after a while he may feel as if he has to keep giving her orgasms, as if nothing will satisfy her. Gradually, sex can become a time-consuming duty for both men and women and lose its magic charm.

Sometimes women in my seminars have told me that they are multiorgasmic, but after ten or so orgasms, they still want more. When they finish sex and the man has his orgasm, the woman doesn't feel satisfied. This is dissatisfying not only for her but for the man as well. He wants to feel that he has given her the ultimate orgasm or at least fulfilled her hunger.

If a woman is generally multiorgasmic, I suggest that instead of having lots of orgasms, she have one big orgasm. She can signal her partner right before her orgasm so that he can lessen stimulation and build her back up. If he builds her up several times, when she finally does have an orgasm, she may happily find that one *is* enough, and she doesn't feel a hunger for more. She is truly satisfied.

Now, when I talk about what works for great sex, I run the risk of sounding as if one approach is the best approach. This is a very male attitude. Men like to find a formula and stick to it. While consistently using one approach may work for men, it generally doesn't work for women. In the next chapter, we will explore the differences between mechanical sex and spontaneous sex.

CHAPTER 10

Mechanical Sex Versus Spontaneous Sex

Another secret of great sex is variety. Women want sex to be a little different every time. Men don't instinctively understand this because they are so goal-oriented. A man seeks to find a formula that will get him where he wants to go, and if it works once, he tends to repeat it over and over. His guiding principle is "If it ain't broke, don't fix it."

Many men find it frustrating to think that each time they have to risk trying something new. A man wants to find a formula that will work each time so he can relax in sex, feeling confident that he knows what he is doing. He feels comfortable with specific formulas. A woman, however, feels most excited when she doesn't know what he is going to do next. Predictability is a turnoff.

∾

**A woman feels most excited in sex
when she doesn't know what her
partner is going to do next.
Predictability is a turnoff.**

∾

No matter how good a sexual formula is, after it is used a few times in a row, it becomes predictable, routine, and eventually boring. When a man is touching her body, unless she is at a peak moment of stimulation, the same stroke over and over can become a little boring. Shifting rhythms and movements may seem unimportant to a man, but to a woman it makes a big difference.

∾

**Shifting rhythms and movements
may seem unimportant to a man,
but to a woman it makes
a big difference.**

∾

Variation in the movement of the body also helps to arouse her more. Sometimes he can lie on top of her, sometimes she can be on top. Sometimes they can switch sides. All this movement helps her to stop thinking and just feel the sensations. While following his lead, she doesn't question why he is gently moving her from time to time, because she feels the thrill of wondering, "Where are we going next?" This anticipation is very exciting to a woman.

❧ Sex and Baseball

To convey a sense of what excites women in sex in terms that most men can really understand, I compare sex to baseball. When a man watches a baseball game, it is the anticipation of what will happen that makes it most exciting. Who will get on base? Will the ball be caught? Who will strike out? Who will score, and who will win?

While he watches the game, his tension builds and releases with every inning. Each time a player gets on base, he feels increasing excitement and tension. This tension is released with hoots of enthusiasm when his team's player moves to another base or scores.

No matter how exciting a game is the first time, if you watch a recording of the exact same game over and over, it will become predictable and boring. In a similar way, when a man follows the same formula in sex, it becomes boring and predictable to his partner.

Sometimes a man will find a formula that

works in sex and change it by making it more efficient. Instead of taking the time for foreplay, he skips ahead to intercourse. This is like tuning in the sports report to find out who won, instead of watching the game itself. Briefly seeing the highlights of a game in a sports summary is certainly fun, but it doesn't come close to the building excitement of being there or watching the whole game.

Watching the entire game makes the conclusion much more exciting. In a similar way, foreplay makes sex very exciting to a woman. It is not just scoring that makes her happy, but the buildup as well.

∽ First Batter Up

To carry the metaphor further, when a man begins gently stroking his forefinger above her breast in foreplay, it is like first batter up. Then, as he begins to move closer to the breast, he hits a line drive. The crowd is excited. She wonders, "Will he get on base?" Then as he approaches her breast, he teases her by pulling back and starting over. Our first batter is out of there, and the crowd moans. Suddenly, the thrill of anticipation arises again as the next batter steps up to the plate.

This time, instead of repeating the stroking motion the same way, he can use two fingers instead of one. This little shift will increase her excitement. It is like having another batter come up. Will he get on base?

Eventually, as he builds up the stimulation, he may be touching one of her breasts, kissing the other. Then he might slowly move his other hand to a different part of her body. Having all this happen gradually is as exciting as having a tie game, with two outs in the ninth inning, bases loaded, and a new batter up. Then when he scores a home run at intercourse, the crowd goes wild as four runs are scored in one play.

∽ The Magic of Foreplay

If he remembers this example of baseball and sex, foreplay will take on a whole new dimension for a man. He can begin to truly understand why foreplay is so important to her.

She has three major erogenous zones to remind a man that there is not just one "point." Her three major zones are also good reminders for him to use both his hands and his mouth.

When using his hand, sometimes he can use one finger, sometimes three. Sometimes he can trace over her body with straight lines and sometimes with wiggly lines. Sometimes his touch can be strong and firm, sometimes extra gentle. Sometimes he may circle his fingers to the right, and then he can go to the left. He can go up and down. Every little variation fulfills her need for variety.

✍

**Every little variation in his touch fulfills
a woman's need for variety.**

✍

By taking the time for foreplay, he increases her pleasure. Don't forget that, as a general rule, a woman needs about ten times more foreplay than a man. As a man gets older, he may need a little more foreplay to become fully aroused, while a woman may sometimes require less. As a general guideline, a man should remember that it is not what he does but how long he takes to do it that ensures her fulfillment.

✍

**A man should remember that it is not
what he does but how long he takes
to do it that ensures
a woman's fulfillment.**

✍

❧

If foreplay has lasted thirty minutes and she hasn't gotten close to orgasm, it's probably safe to say she is not going to have one. Sometimes, however, if he keeps going longer, she will have one. To assist a man in knowing what to do, it is very helpful for a woman to give him some clear feedback.

❧

To assist a man in knowing what to do, it is very helpful for a woman to give him some clear feedback.

❧

If it seems as if he has been stimulating her for a long time and the result is not in sight but she really wants him to continue, she can say something like:

"I really like this a lot."

"I know it's taking a long time, but this really feels good."

> "I don't want this to be over yet. I am loving it."

Also, if he is touching her body and she just needs to silently soak it up and melt into his touch, he may not realize this and begin to panic because he thinks nothing is happening. She can help tremendously by making a comment like:

> "I know I'm really quiet, but I really like this."

> "I really like what you are doing. It is helping me to relax and begin to really open up."

> "Oh, this is just what I needed."

With a little reassuring comment like this, he can keep going without worry that he is doing the wrong things. He needs her positive feedback.

❧

With a little reassuring comment from her, a man can keep going without worry that he is doing the wrong things.

❧

❧ How a Man Can Become More Spontaneous

As we have discussed, it is hard for some men to relax in sex without being able to rely on a formula. A man can solve this problem by having lots of formulas that he rotates using. His favorite pat formula will work if at other times he uses other formulas.

In this way, a man can use formulas but at the same time give the woman the variety she needs. As he picks and chooses from a variety of patterns and skills, she gets to wonder what he is going to do next, and he gets to feel secure that he knows what to do. By alternating techniques in this way, he will automatically begin to create more techniques and approaches. In this way, mechanical sex slowly becomes more and more spontaneous and creative over time.

❧ How a Woman's Sexual Mood Changes

When a man is less mechanical and thus nonpredictable in sex, the woman has the opportunity to explore and express her unique sexual moods or feelings that day. She is more able to be spontaneous and responsive in differing ways. When a woman feels free to change each time, and over time, like the weather, her sexual expression changes. If sex is to remain exciting, her natural changes are important.

∽

∽ Sexual Seasons

Just as the seasons change, so also will sex change and continue to be interesting. For this change to occur naturally, a woman must feel supported in discovering the different expression of her sexual feelings.

The sexual act for a woman is a process of discovering what feels good that day. She does not want her partner to follow any premeditated rigid plan. She would rather that sex be a spontaneous creation each time, appropriate to how both partners are feeling.

This requires a new skill. As we have already discussed, a man instinctively prefers a tried and tested formula because he is then assured that he will fulfill his partner. A woman also wants him to know what to do, but in a different way.

She wants him to know that each time her mood may be different. She wants him to know how to discover with her what she wants. She wants him to be sensitive to her feedback that will assist him in leading her to higher states of fulfillment and pleasure.

To do this, a man needs to know the basics of great sex and to be willing to experiment by rotating his various skills. Like an artist, he needs to be very familiar with the basic colors of sex and then experiment with how they combine to create a new work of art. Like a musician, he needs to know the basic notes and chord combinations to create a beautiful piece of music.

❧

Like an artist, he needs to be very familiar with the basic colors of sex and then experiment with how they combine to create a new work of art.

❧

~ Following His Lead

When a man can take the lead in sex, he frees his partner to think less and feel more. This does not mean that she just lies there passively. The freedom to relax and stop thinking about what "should" happen allows her to flow in the currents and undulating rhythms of her sensual and sexual nature. Like dancing to a particular type of music, she can move and dance with him to the rhythm of her mood that day.

Sometimes she might feel like wrapping up next to his body, entwining him and seducing him with her body. At other times, she might feel like she is experiencing his touch for the first time. Or she might start out cool and reserved but then gradually, as he touches her body, be taken over by passion. She might feel assertive, or she may peacefully cuddle up to him and melt into a deeply relaxing place as he gently touches her. These different expressions of her sexual nature are not planned or thought out, but instead are discovered in the moment.

〜

〜

**Different expressions of her sexual
nature are not planned or thought out,
but instead are discovered
in the moment.**

〜

When a woman has the freedom to be
spontaneous, these different expressions
and others will naturally come up and be expressed. When a man carefully takes the
time to stimulate a woman with no expectations of how she is supposed to respond,
over time she feels safer and safer in sex to
do and express whatever she feels. This un-
inhibited sexual expression frees her to enjoy new sexual experiences.

~ Communicating About Sex

Both men and women need clear and positive feedback to know what brings their
partners the greatest fulfillment. I recommend that you take a half hour sometime,
particularly when you are not feeling negative about sex, and talk about your sexual
experience. In fact, it's a good idea to have
an update on this conversation every few
years in your relationship.

Here is a list of questions to stimulate an
informative conversation.

"What do you like about having sex
with me?"

"How did you feel when I did that?"

"Would you like more sex?"

"About how much sex would you like
each week?"

~

"Would you like more time in foreplay sometimes?"

"Would you like less time in foreplay sometimes?"

"Is there something specific you would like me to do in the next month during sex?"

"Is there a new way you would like me to touch you? If yes, would you show me?"

"Is there anything new you would like me to try?"

"Is there anything you would like to try sexually that we've never done?"

"Is there anything I used to do that you would like me to do more of?"

If you are not having sex or are not completely satisfied, it is OK to have this kind of conversation, but be very careful to put aside any negative feelings, complaints, and criticisms. Talking about sex is very, very delicate.

What makes it difficult to talk about our needs in bed is that we don't want to feel that we are in any way disappointing our partners, but at the same time, we don't want to be expected to do what doesn't feel comfortable or natural to us. When answering these questions, it is important that you make it clear that you are not demanding more.

You should not do things that do not feel right to you. When your partner does not seem open to things you favor, it is critically important to be nonjudgmental and accept your partner's feelings. At the same time, if your partner wants something that doesn't seem important to you or seems unpleasant at first, keep an open mind. You can always say, "At this point, that feels like too big a stretch for me, but I am definitely considering it."

A way to let your partner know something is really important to you is to gently and persistently bring it up in a friendly and nondemanding way each time you occasionally have this kind of conversation about sex. A secret of great sex is to build on the strengths you have and not focus on the problems or what you are missing. Many men and women have shared with me that after hearing my tapes on sex, they were able to automatically release some "prudish" ideas about sex and really begin to enjoy the pleasures of sex with someone they love.

∽

A *secret of great sex is to build on the strengths you have and not focus on the problems or what you are missing.*

∽

In the next chapter, we explore how monogamy helps to keep sex passionate and alive.

CHAPTER 11

Passionate Monogamy

For some people, the thought of having sex with one person all their life seems too boring. They want more excitement. When you learn how to make sex spontaneous and not mechanical, it doesn't have to become boring. Over time the feeling of sex can continue to change and passion can continue to grow.

There is no doubt in my mind that the secret of success in my marriage is the sexual commitment we have to each other. Many men don't realize why monogamy is so important. They don't instinctively understand that monogamy ensures that a woman continues to feel special and loved. If she is not feeling loved in this way, she cannot continue to open herself to him. Trust is essential for a woman to continue getting turned on to her partner.

❧

> **Trust is essential for a woman to continue getting turned on to her partner.**

❧

It is easy for a man to be turned on to a woman he is attracted to. It is not so automatic to keep that attraction. It is not enough for a man to love a woman. He needs to feel that she is attracted to him, that she is open to him. He needs to feel that he can make her happy.

❧

> **A man needs to repeatedly experience that he can make a woman happy if he is to stay attracted and turned on to her.**

❧

~

~ Why Passion Is Easy in the Beginning

In the beginning of a relationship, as she looks into his eyes and then casually looks away, he gets the clear message that he could be the one to make her happy. This look gives him the courage to risk rejection and initiate a relationship.

Later on, when he has disappointed her several times, she stops giving him that look, and he stops feeling that he can make her happy. Suddenly or gradually, the attraction stops. He may love her, but he is no longer attracted to her.

He may fantasize about having sex with other women, or he may eventually just suppress his sexual tendencies. He is still monogamous, but there is no passion. To remain a prisoner in a passionless relationship is not a choice that people today are willing to make. Using advanced relationship skills in bed and out can ensure that passion stays alive and sex continues to get better and better.

∽ The Ebb and Flow of Passion

It is both healthy and natural that the wave of passion in a relationship rises and falls. Just as it is normal not to feel in love with your partner at times, it is also normal not to feel sexually attracted to your partner.

∽

Just as it is normal not to feel in love with your partner at times, it is also normal not to feel sexually attracted to your partner.

∽

Times when you don't feel this sexual attraction are like cloudy days when the sun doesn't shine. A cloudy day does not mean the sun is not there. It just means that it is temporarily covered. Cloudy days are the times when temptation knocks on our doors. When attraction is blocked in a relationship, many times we feel attracted elsewhere.

To maintain the possibility for passion to come back to your relationship, ideally it is best not to indulge your passions or fantasies.

At times, I have found myself getting turned on to another woman. This doesn't mean I don't love my wife. It just means that my attraction is not fully locked in to my wife. It takes years of commitment before a man's passions flow only in the direction of his partner.

~ When a Man Is Tempted

When I am turned on to another woman, I look down at myself and think, "I'm glad everything down there is working." Then I point in the opposite direction and say, "Home, James."

I never tell myself I'm bad for feeling attracted to someone else, but I take that arousal and bring it back to my wife. If I get home and it is gone, I know I just have to be-

〜

gin using my advanced relationship skills to make her feel loved, happy, and special. Gradually, the attraction always comes back.

Just by containing my sexual feelings and repeatedly directing them to my wife, I increase my ability to be turned on to her. Also by controlling my feelings when I am away from her, I have more control in sex.

〜 When a Man Can Control His Passion

When a man can both feel his passion and control it, a woman can begin to let go of control, release her inhibitions, and start to really feel her passions. As a man learns to control his passions, not only does he help his partner reach higher levels of fulfillment, but he also can experience greater levels of sexual pleasure and love.

～

～

When a man can feel his passion and control it, a woman can begin to let go of control, release her inhibitions, and start to really feel her passions.

～

When a man is in control, it means that his passion is so great that he could easily have an orgasm, but instead he holds back and gradually builds up his partner's passion.

～ The Importance of Monogamy for Great Sex

This control is not exercised just in bed but extends into the world. When a man is in touch with his sexual feelings but directs his sexual energies only to his partner, this control has a definite effect on her.

Every time a man is tempted by the possibility of sex and maintains his monogamous commitment, he is creating the safety for his partner to enjoy sex more. By not indulging in his fantasies of other women, he learns to control his sexual energies so that he can slow down the process of release and last longer for her. Certainly, thoughts and images may cross his mind, but as long as he comes back to an awareness of his partner, his passion and control will continue to grow.

Some men can easily last long but have little passion. Other men have tremendous excitement and passion but little control. Once they get started, they are quickly finished. They experience sexual release, but it is not as good as it could be. Using the skills of polarity sex can help a man last longer, but through years of passionate monogamy, he will automatically find more control.

᠅ How a Woman Can Help a Man Last Longer

Just as a man affects a woman's ability to relinquish control and enjoy the moment, a woman's trust and ability to open up and receive from his touch and love can help a man stay in control.

When a woman is able to surrender and fully receive a man, he can easily maintain control while feeling increasing passion. When she is able to relax, receive, and enjoy his loving touch, he can last longer. He can continue giving as long as she is fully receiving.

If, however, she tries to take control and start turning him on, she can unknowingly push him out of control or turn him off. When he is focused on giving to her and arousing her, but she is trying to turn him on rather than let him turn her on, she can actually block the flow of his energy into her and cause him to have an orgasm before he is ready.

When her sexual reactions are a response

to him rather than an attempt to arouse him, he can grow in controlled passion. But when her responses are not genuine reactions to his skillful touch, he doesn't feel the growth of passion and may suddenly lose control. He either gets too excited or he gets turned off. In both cases, he doesn't know what happened, nor does she. By her being overly excited to his touch in this manner, she can actually turn him off.

❧ Repeating the Fourth of July

One afternoon, Donald and Connie had great, fantastic, memorable sex. Afterward, Donald told her how much he loved it. He felt that she had truly enjoyed the moment, and he was happy she had freely expressed her passion.

Two days later when they were having sex, right away she began making the same moves from the time before. This time it was

a turnoff for him, even though she was repeating what she had done before to please
him.

He didn't understand at first what had
gone wrong. Then he realized that the previous time when he had liked it so much, her
movements were spontaneous. The next
time, she was mechanically doing it, and
that is why it didn't work. Her passionate
movements and feelings were not an automatic response to him but instead were her
loving attempt to please him again.

Quite innocently, she was just doing what
she knew he had liked before. After dis-
cussing this, Connie learned that her honest
and natural expression would turn Donald
on the best, particularly when he was trying
to turn her on. This awareness freed her to
look even more deeply to her authentic sexual responses.

Balancing Her Pleasure with His

When a man finds himself about to have an orgasm before she is ready, he can easily regain control by reducing his excitement and increasing hers. By focusing his attention on her and not letting her focus on giving more pleasure to him, he can begin to increase her pleasure. As she begins to receive more pleasure than he does, his control comes back.

Choosing to Slow Down

Sometimes a man feels that once intercourse has begun, if he is a real man he should maintain a constant rhythm. Quite the opposite is true. A woman appreciates that she can turn a man on so that he begins to lose control. This is a turn-on for her. When he needs to pause for a moment, she feels successful in exciting him and she feels he is considerate of her. His slowing down to pace his energy and pleasure with hers is a sign of great skill and control and has the effect of increasing her pleasure.

Without an understanding of how she feels, he may feel inadequate and out of control because he can't continue his rhythm. She, however, will feel happy that he is in so much control that he can slow down for her.

If he is so aroused that he can't continue intercourse without having an orgasm before she does, he should just slow down and either lie quietly for a few minutes to calm down or gently pull out and continue stimulating her.

Whenever he is starting to lose control, it is generally a sign that she can't keep up. Sometimes to seem as if she is keeping up, she will intensify her passion, hoping to please him or catch up. At this point, he will tend to lose control and climax too soon. Neither he nor she feels very good when this happens.

Mistakes do happen, and certainly we should never expect sex to be "perfect" each time. When a man does occasionally climax before a woman, instead of feeling bad, he can just make a mental note to make sure that next time he gives her an orgasm before he has his.

He might playfully say:

"I owe you one, honey."

"You were just too irresistible tonight, next time I'll make sure you get yours."

"I love you sweetheart, next time will be all for you."

After this, it's best not to talk much about it but just behave as if everything is fine. If he seems disappointed and moody, the best thing she can do is to act as if everything is fine and leave him alone for a while. If, however, she is disappointed and feels a need to have an orgasm right away, she can simply begin bringing herself to climax while he holds her or helps.

~ When a Man Doesn't Get an Erection

Just as a man may easily lose control, he may also not get an erection right away. As a rule of thumb, in both cases the solution is the same. He should focus more on her pleasure. As her pleasure increases and she lets go of control, he regains his control. Couples generally make the mistake of focusing on him as if he has a problem. The more the woman focuses on trying to give him an erection, the more difficult it becomes.

~

*When a man doesn't get an erection or
has difficulty maintaining control,
he should simply focus
more on her pleasure.*

~

Although sometimes it can be helpful to see a counselor for assistance, it is best to first ignore a man's lack of control when it occurs and focus on ways he can help her feel loved in the relationship. Then when it comes to sex, they can both focus on her fulfillment for a while without depending on his erection.

A tremendous amount of pleasure can be shared sexually without a man having to be erect. The best solution is generally to focus on what techniques he can use to skillfully turn her on. Automatically, his erections will then begin to come back.

Although it is important not to be mechanical in sex, it is also important to understand in very concrete terms the basic mechanics of sex. In the next chapter, we will explore our different sexual anatomies and different ways to successfully stimulate each other.

CHAPTER 12

Sexual Anatomy

Because stimulation of the woman's genitals is so important for a woman's fulfillment, I would like to take a moment to review some basic terms about a woman's anatomy. The term "vulva" describes all the female external genital organs, including the labia majora, the labia minora, the clitoris, and the entrance to the vagina.

The labia majora are outside the labia minora, which are the smaller folds of flesh inside the external folds. Both sets of folds contain thousands of delicate nerve fibers running up and down, which, when delicately stroked, provide much stimulation, pleasure, and fulfillment.

At the south end of the labia is the vagina,

which is the canal where the man enters her body. At the north end of the labia is the clitoris. Because it is so small and because he does not have one, a man doesn't realize how important it is to a woman for him to touch her there. As a general rule, it is very important for a man to remember to go north before he goes south.

❧

**It is very important for a man
to remember to go north before
he goes south.**

❧

When a woman is very aroused, a man can stimulate her even more intensely by pressing a couple of fingers just north of the clitoris and then pulling back. This, however, should be done cautiously. If this sensitive area is touched with too much pressure or too soon, even if she is in the mood for an orgasm, she may not be able to have one.

Too much pressure can temporarily numb her sensations.

Men should aim to have a feather touch down there. When the woman wants it harder, she can easily let him know.

~ Camping Out "Down South"

While touching a woman's genitals, a man needs to remember to vary his approach from time to time. Instead of using the same finger, try another one. Then use two, then three. Occasionally use the whole palm as you gently but firmly sweep up from the south to the north.

Sometimes it is good to grab a pillow and plan to camp out down south for a full fifteen minutes. You should just resign yourself to the fact that you are not going anywhere else for quite a while. In this relaxed way, you can experiment.

Try moving with the rhythm of her breathing. As she becomes more excited, increase the pace. Then slow down. Increase and decrease, no hurry, nowhere to go. A variety of movements without rhyme or reason can be very stimulating for her.

While using different movements, you should listen to her responses to know what is working best that day and do more of it. Play with the movement. Do variations of it, and then come back to it. Even a winning movement can become boring if it is used too much. Yet once she is very excited, keeping a steady and consistent movement can assist her in reaching higher levels of pleasure.

❦

Once she is very excited, keeping a steady and consistent movement can assist her in reaching higher levels of pleasure.

❦

෴

෴ Camping Out "Down South" for Women

Pleasing a man "down South" is one of the few ways she can directly give her love to him. It can be a beautiful gift of her love for him.

There are two basic ways to stimulate the penis: friction and compression. Friction is generated by rubbing up and down, and compression is created by holding the penis and squeezing and releasing.

Sometimes she can move slow and then speed up. While moving up and down, she can also use her other hand and grip the penis around its base.

She can use the basic up and down movement quickly without a lot of pressure. This fast movement can actually help him to control his pleasure better because it is less intense than intercourse.

If she wants to increase the intensity, she can squeeze tighter as she moves up and down. Different varied movements and grips provide increasing stimulation for him but also fun for her.

❧ Spreading Out the Pleasure

Once she has stimulated his penis for a while, the rest of his body becomes much more sensuous. To increase his pleasure, she can then begin to spread the pleasure out around his body.

Just as a man needs feedback, so does a woman. When she is doing something that he really likes, it is OK for him to say, "I really like that movement." Various sounds of pleasure can also let her know what he likes most.

By using a variety of pressures and alternating between intense movement and light movement, a woman can build his energy up and then let it settle down. Each time she builds his energy back up, his pleasure will be greater.

Just as a woman stimulating a man's penis is very exciting and important to him, romance is exciting to women. When she is stimulating him, a man gets to relax and be loved at a time when he is most vulnerable. It is his time to receive, after all his efforts to give. Similarly, romance is a way a man can give to a woman and let her know that he loves her and appreciates her efforts.

In the next chapter, we will explore different rituals for lasting romance.

CHAPTER 13

Keeping the Magic of Magic of Romance Alive

While men hunger for great sex, women long for romance. Even the tough-minded, goal-oriented, high-powered executive woman places great value on romance. Romance has a magical effect on women everywhere.

Women spend billions of dollars each year on romance novels. To fulfill a woman's need for romance, a man first needs to understand what romance is. Receiving cards, cut flowers and little presents; moonlit nights; spontaneous decisions; and eating out all spell romance.

It is not that men are unwilling to create romance. A man just doesn't get why it is so important. He is happy to be romantic in the beginning to show her how special she is, but once he has behaved romantically, he doesn't instinctively realize why he has to keep doing it. Probably if he had repeatedly witnessed his father being romantic to his mother, it wouldn't have to be a learned skill.

❧ The Magic of Cut Flowers

I remember once asking my wife to pick up some flowers at the grocery store. I knew that women like cut flowers, but after a while I wondered why I should keep getting them. After all, I casually thought, she could easily pick them up while she was shopping.

To her, this kind of reasoning was definitely not romantic. Through eventually discovering the importance of buying her cut flowers, I was able to understand the importance of all romantic gestures.

To feel romanced, a woman doesn't want to buy her own flowers. She wants her lover to do it. She doesn't even want to ask for them. If she has to ask, it doesn't count as romance.

His self-motivated purchase of cut flowers for her is a symbol that he cares for her and understands her needs. These kinds of symbols are a very important part of romance.

❧

His self-motivated purchase of cut flowers for her is a symbol that he cares for her and understands her needs.

❧

She does not want a potted plant but cut flowers that will die in five days. Why cut flowers? So that in five days he will again go out and prove his love for her by purchasing more flowers!

Buying a potted plant is just not romantic. It is one more thing she will have to take care of.

∽ How a Woman Can Help Him Be Romantic

When I forget to buy flowers, Bonnie sometimes helps me to remember. Instead of buying them herself or asking me to buy them, she will put out empty vases. In this way, I get to notice and then take full credit for bringing them home.

Not only do I feel charming and dashing, but she gets to feel more fully that I care. If she puts out the vases and I still forget, instead of buying flowers herself, she will sometimes ask me.

Although it is not as romantic, she can then appreciate the flowers and I will feel closer to her because I did get them. Once again, after I experience how happy the flowers make her, I tend to remember to buy them.

∽ Why Romance Works

When a man plans a date, handles the tickets, drives the car, and takes care of all the small details, that is romance. When a man takes responsibility to take care of things, it allows a woman to relax and enjoy feeling taken care of. It is like a mini vacation that assists her to come back to her female side.

∽

Romance is like a mini vacation that assists her in coming back to her female side.

∽

Romantic moments are particularly helpful for women who don't feel comfortable sharing their feelings. On a romantic date, without having to talk about her feelings, a woman can feel acknowledged, adored, understood, and supported. She receives the benefits of talking without having to talk.

A man's romantic behavior says repeatedly that he acknowledges her, and by anticipating her needs, he signals that he understands and respects her. These kinds of actions give her the same support that talking does. In both cases, she feels heard.

❧ Why Romance Is Important

Romance is so important today because it assists a woman to come back to her female side. For most of the day, she is doing a traditionally male job that requires her to move more to her male side. To find relief, she needs her partner's help to return to her female side.

Romance clearly places the woman in the feminine role of being special and cared for. When a man passionately focuses on fulfilling her needs, she is able to release her tendency to take care of others. For romance to stay alive, however, eventually there must be good communication.

∽

∽ Romance and Communication

For romance to thrive, a woman needs to feel heard and understood on a day-to-day basis. In the beginning of a relationship, the woman really doesn't know the man and can imagine that she is truly seen, understood, and validated. This positive feeling is the fertile ground of romance and passion. After several disappointments, however, this magic spell is broken.

When the man is untrained in the skills of listening to and understanding a woman, or when the woman resists sharing the feelings that naturally come up, she eventually feels unheard and is turned off. She generally doesn't even know what happened. He may even make romantic overtures, but they don't have the same magical feeling. Even cut flowers lose their potency if a woman doesn't feel heard on a daily basis.

Talking is a major feminine need. I fully develop this advanced relationship skill in my other books on relationships and communication. Creating romantic rituals that say, "I love you and I care about you" can, however, go a long way to communicate love without words. With the support of romance, communication is much easier.

✎ Creating Romantic Rituals

In my relationship with Bonnie, we have several rituals that nurture her female side while supporting my male side. Romantic rituals are simple actions that acknowledge he cares about her and she appreciates him. Here's an example.

✎

Romantic rituals are simple actions that acknowledge he cares about her and she appreciates him.

✎

∽

As a writer, I have an office in my home. When I hear her come home during the day, I immediately stop, get up, and find her. I greet her with a hug. Like bringing flowers, this little ritual creates a feeling that I care about her and she is loved. When she lights up after I greet her in this way, I also feel loved and appreciated.

If I forget to greet her, she will find me, not always right away, and greet me by asking me for a hug and then really appreciating it.

For many women, the thought of having to ask for a hug seems paradoxical. A hug makes her feel supported. To have to ask for a hug affirms that she is not supported. Certainly, it is more romantic if the man offers to give the hug, but if he forgets, it is better to ask than to miss out and be resentful.

∽

It is more romantic if the man offers
to give the hug, but if he forgets,
it is better to ask than to
miss out and be resentful.

∽

∽ **Asking for Love: The Big Step**

I remember when Bonnie first asked for a
hug. It made such a difference in our relationship. Instead of resenting me for not offering hugs, she would simply ask.

It was such a gift of love to me. She began
to understand that the way to love me best
was to help me be successful in loving her.
This is a very important advanced relationship skill.

I still remember the first day she asked for
a hug. I was standing in my closet, and she
was making different sounds of exhaustion.
She said, "Ooohhh, what a day."

⤙

Then she took a deep breath and made a long sigh on the exhale. In her language, she was asking for a hug. What I heard was a tired person and wrongly assumed that she probably wanted to be left alone.

Instead of resenting me for not noticing or responding to her request, she took the big step to ask for what she wanted, even though to her it seemed obvious.

She said, "John, would you give me a hug?"

My response was immediate. I said, "Of course." I went straight over to her and gave her a big hug.

She let out another big sigh in my arms and then thanked me for the hug. I said, "Any time."

She chuckled and smiled. I said, "What?"

She said, "You have no idea how hard it was to ask for a hug."

I said, "Really? Why should it be hard? I am always willing to give you a hug, if you want one."

She said, "I know, but it feels so humiliating to have to ask. I feel like I am begging for love. I want to feel like you want to give me a hug as much as I want one. I have this romantic picture that you will notice that I need a hug, then automatically offer one."

I said, "Oh . . . well, from now on I will definitely try to notice and offer to give you hugs. And I really thank you for asking. If I forget to notice in the future, I hope you will keep asking."

❧ Acknowledge Her When She Seems Distant

Just this morning, I noticed a little distance from my wife. Instead of giving her a lot of space or ignoring her, I immediately asked her how she was feeling. This is another important ritual.

I said, "Are you feeling OK?"

Bonnie said, "I am feeling a little lonely, like the wife of an author."

Instead of taking this as an invitation for an argument regarding how much time I spend on writing versus on our relationship, I heard what she was really saying. She was just feeling lonely. She didn't mean anything more except that she would love a hug. So instead of defending myself, I said emphatically, "Ohhh, come here . . . let me give you a hug."

෨ Eating Out

This same principle of asking for what you want applies to all romantic rituals. When Cindy is tired, her husband, Bob, offers either to make dinner or to take her out. If he doesn't notice or offer, she will ask, "Bob, would you take us out to eat tonight?" or "Bob, would you pick up something to go and bring it home for dinner?" or "Bob, would you make dinner tonight?"

The flip side of this ritual is that when they are finished eating out, Cindy always thanks Bob for a wonderful meal. Even though it is *their* money that pays for the meal, she thanks him. If he brings home food, she appreciates it in the same way as when he makes a meal.

❧ Ordering the Meal

Another little ritual while eating out is for the man to ask the woman what she is going to order and then order it for her when the waiter arrives. Although a man need not always do this, when he does, it makes dinner special. It gives her the message that he is attentive to her, he remembers what she likes, and he cares.

When he orders for her, it does not imply that she can't order for herself. His ordering for her is just a romantic ritual that says, "You are always doing so much for me and others, so let me do this for you."

Another way to create a little romance in the restaurant is for him to suggest things that he knows she likes. This increases her feeling that she is seen, heard, and known.

Ironically, if she suggests foods for him to eat, he may feel as if she is mothering him, which is not romantic. What may be romantic for her is not romantic for him.

~ How Men Take Credit

One way a woman can create some romance when they eat out is simply to have a good time and appreciate the food or the restaurant. When he takes her out, on an emotional level he will tend to take credit for the dinner. If she likes the dinner, he feels, "Yes, I cooked that dinner."

When a man takes a woman out, she has a golden opportunity to make him feel special as well. When she appreciates what he provides for her, he feels more intimate with her.

When a man and woman go to a movie and she likes the movie, then again, a part of him takes credit. He feels, "Yes, I wrote that movie, I directed it, and I starred in it." Of course, intellectually he knows he didn't create the movie, but emotionally it is as if he did.

To keep the romance, she can be sensitive to his feelings when she is not happy with a movie. She doesn't need to point out to him in great detail that she didn't like the movie. A man feels most romantic when he feels successful in providing for her happiness.

↩ Focusing on the Good

Sometimes a man will sense that she didn't like the movie and for reassurance ask, "Did you like the movie?" He doesn't really want an accurate answer about the movie but some nice and friendly comment so that he doesn't feel he ruined the evening.

To support him at those vulnerable and embarrassing times, she needs to focus on the positive and look for something that was good or that she appreciated. She could pause for a while to let him know that she is working hard to find something good about the movie. The longer she takes, the more he knows she didn't like the movie, and the more he'll appreciate her for not complaining about it. After pausing to find something that she liked, she can still be honest but not critical. She could say, "I really liked that sunset scene. That was beautiful photography."

Even if there was absolutely nothing good about it, she could say, "I don't think I have ever seen a movie like that." He will get the message right away and change the subject.

Or she could say, "I just enjoyed being with you." He will definitely appreciate her.

She will find it easier to make the effort to give these kinds of supportive comments when she understands that he is really asking for her to help him save face.

Just as little gifts and caring attention from a man to a woman make her feel loved and romantic, when a woman appreciates a man's efforts and what he provides for her, he feels more loved and romantically inclined.

It is attention to the little things that creates lasting romance. When men and women take each other for granted, the romance disappears.

ᴖ Some Things Are Better Left Unsaid

Once in my seminar, while sharing this example about reacting to a movie, a woman said, "It just doesn't feel honest to me to do that. Why can't I just tell him?"

I said, "I can understand your frustration, but to help you understand the situation better, let me ask you a question."

She smiled and nodded her head.

I said, "What should a man say when his wife is getting dressed and looking into the mirror and says, 'Do you think I am getting fat?' " She immediately began to laugh and said she got the message.

When it comes to romance, there are just some things better left unsaid, particularly at sensitive moments. The reason men and women tend to be insensitive is that they do not instinctively understand their different sensitivities. A man might think, "Why do I have to keep bringing her flowers or opening doors for her?" and a woman might think, "Why do I have to acknowledge the things he does?" As we understand each other better, these little rituals become fun and playful, and, most important, they are loving, kind, and considerate.

❧

As we understand each other better, these little rituals become fun and playful, and, most important, they are loving, kind, and considerate.

❧

∽ Survival Skills for Dating

If a woman doesn't understand this delicate point, while dating she can easily turn her partner off without even realizing it.

Here is another example. Bonnie and I were going to see a really great movie. We both loved it. But what I remember even more clearly than the movie was the comment a woman made on her way out to her date.

He had just asked her if she liked the movie. She responded that she hated it. I watched his posture droop as he then said, "What would you like to do now?"

She said, "I'd like to stand outside this theater and tell every person how awful this movie was." I still remember the defeated look in this fellow's eyes.

This woman didn't even have a clue that she was destroying whatever chance of romance they had that evening. This man was definitely going to hesitate before ever picking another movie with her again.

∽ Telling the Truth

Telling the truth in a relationship is essential for intimacy and romance to thrive, but timing is equally important. Lasting romance requires talking at the right time and in a way that doesn't offend, hurt, or sour your partner.

∽

Telling the truth in a relationship is essential for intimacy and romance to thrive, but timing is equally important.

∽

Having lots of successful romantic rituals gives both men and women the emotional support they need to be more honest, particularly about the important things. When a man feels appreciated, it is easier for him to hear and respond lovingly to her feelings and needs. When he doesn't feel appreciated and hears her talk about problems, he feels as if she is saying he is not doing enough.

∼

Having lots of successful romantic rituals gives both men and women the emotional support they need to be more honest, particularly about the important things.

∼

Listening to a woman's feelings is a new skill for men. Traditionally, men have *not* been expected to empathetically listen to women's feelings. If a woman was upset, he would "do something" or "fix something" to make her feel better. When a woman needed empathy, to get emotional support, she didn't talk to a man, she went to other women. Until recently, women didn't even want to talk with men about their feelings.

༄ Why Talking Helps Romance

Today women don't have time for each other. To various degrees, they are all feeling overwhelmed with too much to do. Lacking the support of other women *and* having to talk in a very goal-oriented way at work, many women today are not merely hungry to share their feelings at the end of the day, but starving. In a magical way, this new dilemma can actually be a terrific opportunity for romance.

As we have discussed before, men need to feel needed and appreciated. This is their primary emotional fuel. A big problem arises when women can provide for and protect themselves. In a very real way, men are out of work; they have been laid off from the job they have exclusively held for thousands of years.

Although women are no longer as dependent on men as providers and protectors, they suddenly have a new emerging need: a man to talk to; a partner who truly cares and listens. Women today need to communicate and feel heard at the end of the day.

∽ The Importance of Communication

Sometimes even before she can appreciate romantic gestures, a woman needs to communicate and feel heard. Just as sex connects a man to his feelings, communication connects a woman to her need for and appreciation of romance.

∽

Just as sex connects a man to his feelings, communication connects a woman to her need for and appreciation of romance.

∽

For the last twenty years, the lack of communication in intimate relationships has been the major complaint of women. The reason for this is simple: Overworked women need to talk more about their feelings to successfully cope with the stress of being overwhelmed.

☙

Overworked women need to talk more about their feelings to successfully cope with the stress of being overwhelmed.

☙

By learning to fulfill this new emerging need to talk with his mate, a man is back in the saddle and able to provide for his partner in a new and equally important way. By gradually learning to listen, a man helps a woman be released from feeling overwhelmed and gives her a reason to greatly appreciate him.

❧ Opening the Car Door

Romantic rituals or habits are ways the truth of your deepest feelings can be easily expressed. Opening the car is another of those rituals. Particularly for men, doing such things is a way of showing love. When a woman appreciates his efforts, not only does he feel closer to her, but her heart begins to open as well.

❧

*Romantic rituals or habits
are ways the truth of your
deepest feelings can be
easily expressed.*

❧

When a couple goes out on a date, he should go to her side of the car and open the door—even if the car automatically unlocks with a little beeper. If he starts forgetting to do this, she can remind him the next time as they approach the car by simply wrapping her arm inside his so he naturally escorts her to the door.

Even if he is opening the door for her, the very feminine act of cuddling next to her man and wrapping her arm around him is very nurturing both for her and for him.

✌ Write It Down

Another romantic ritual is to write down a request. When a woman asks for something and he can't give her an immediate response, the next best thing is for her to see him write it down. If he doesn't write it down, she feels that she will have to remember and remind him again and again. A woman feels romanced by a man who hears her and quickly addresses her requests or at least writes them down. This kind of immediate response gives her the feeling that he is really there for her. Just as men like women to respond in sex, women like men to respond to little requests.

> *Just as men like women to respond in sex, women like men to respond to little requests.*

Whenever possible, if her request can be met immediately in just a couple of minutes, the best way to ensure lasting romance is for him to "do it now." A quick response is so comforting for a woman. When she says, for example, "The lightbulb upstairs went out," he can think, "That only takes two minutes, do it now," and then say, "I'll change it right now." Before I understood that it was the little things that make a big difference with women, I would have just put it on the bottom of my to-do list because other lights were working. I would not have gotten around to doing it until much later.

The truth is it only takes two minutes for a man to get a lightbulb and screw it in. When a woman makes a little request like this, a smart man immediately responds, and she loves it.

I don't want to imply that men should just stand around waiting to do whatever she wants. Of course, men can be very busy or very tired, and they need to do things for themselves just as they do things for her. If she says the yard is a mess, he doesn't have to jump up and start working on it. That kind of request takes hours to fulfill. It can go on the "to be done later" list.

Just as a man needs to listen and respond to her needs and requests in whatever way he can, a woman's way of creating romance is to not take anything he does for her for granted. Certainly, there will be times that she doesn't respond with appreciation, just as there will be times when he doesn't respond immediately to her requests, but by being aware of these basic dynamics at work, they will always be moving in the right direction.

As couples practice keeping romance alive, it actually gets easier and easier. When a man anticipates he will be appreciated for doing something, he has more energy to do it. When a woman anticipates he will hear her and respond, she feels much more appreciative and can more easily acknowledge all he does and be more forgiving at those times when he makes mistakes or seems self-centered or lazy.

When a woman consistently lets a man know what a great guy he is for the little things he does, he will continue to do them. It brings out the best in him. Without her support, he will probably unconsciously go back to focusing on the big things like making money and being a good provider. When he does little things for her, it gives her the chance to feel her love for him again and again. She may love him, but if he doesn't do things for her, it is also hard for her to feel her romantic feelings for him.

Rituals take time to develop, but each time a man gets into the habit of doing something a woman likes, and she continues to express her appreciation instead of taking it for granted, he will automatically be motivated to do a little more.

⤳ Going for a Walk Together

One of Robert and Cher's romantic rituals is to walk together. Cher loves to go for walks. In the beginning of the relationship, Robert was more of a workaholic. When Cher asked him if he wanted to go for a walk, he would say no because he needed to work.

One day, he realized that a walk only takes about fifteen minutes, and since Cher loved to walk, it would probably be very good for their relationship. He remembered that when she was upset, she would say things like, "We are so busy, we never have time for each other."

As an experiment, he started taking little walks with her. In the beginning, he didn't get much out of it, but now he loves it. At first, they would walk and she would talk.

His mind was rather distracted by the pressures of work. She easily could have gotten upset that he was thinking about work the whole time, but instead she wisely enjoyed being with him, without expecting anything more from him. Cher was content to talk about how beautiful the trees were.

Gradually because it was something that made her happy, he began to like it more and more. Now he goes for walks even when she is not around. He likes it. It is a great break, and when he comes back he is more relaxed, clear, and efficient.

Our Night Out

Philip and Lori make sure that at least one night a week, they go out and have fun without feeling the pressures of their home and family. Sometimes, of course, they go out several times, but they always go out on Tuesday night.

Tuesday night is their movie night. They

both love movies. Then every other week they will additionally do something more cultural like attending the theater or a concert.

These kinds of little rituals are particularly important for women because they give them an inner sense of security that they will get the special emotional support they need from a relationship to cope with the stress of daily life.

∾ Going Out With the Guys

Each week, Craig has a ritual of going to the movies or doing something with his male friends. They generally go and see a "guy" movie, the kind of movie his wife, Sarah, doesn't like.

Although at first this kind of ritual may not seem to support their relationship, it really does. Spending time with the guys keeps him from expecting to get all his support from Sarah. Time away helps him to feel completely free to be himself. As a result, he begins to miss her and want to be with her even more.

Sarah understands this because she greatly appreciates the support he gives her to spend time with her women friends. He recognizes that it is vitally important for her to get many of her needs met by women friends so that she is not looking to him for everything.

When he goes out with the guys, her accepting attitude about it really makes him feel her support. It used to be that she would look at him in a hurt way whenever he went out with the guys. Now she even reminds him to go out when he forgets.

〜 **Building Fires**

Charley and Carol have a ritual around building fires. In the wintertime, when Charley got cold he used to just go turn up the heater. Now instead he will find his wife first and ask her if she is cold. Just including her in that way makes her feel special.

When he wants to create more romance, he will offer to build a fire. There is something very special when a man builds a fire for a woman. Certain primal feelings are awakened. There is a good reason that so many resorts have fireplaces in the bedrooms.

When they first moved into their forest home, Carol was planning to make lots of changes. Charley thought they were all good ideas. As he continued to support her ideas, he kept thinking of what he would want.

He wanted one of those automatic fireplaces that burns gas. When a switch was turned, it would automatically light, and the fire was all ready. Carol, however, was not into high-tech fireplaces.

When he suggested it, in a positive way she said, "That sounds like a good idea. I can see why you would want that."

After a pause, he started thinking, "OK, she's going to go for it."

Then she said, "I don't know. Something very special happens inside me when you build me a fire. It is very primal." Because he understood the power of these romantic rituals, he gave up on the idea of the high-tech fireplace and is now glad he did.

All it takes sometimes to create a special romantic mood at home is for him to build a fire. He will wait till she is home and then carry in the heavy logs. Then he will sit down and begin building the fire.

She appreciates every effort he makes. It is special for her to feel that he is taking care of her. Sometimes she will build a fire herself, and although it is nice, it doesn't automatically kindle the fires of their romantic feelings.

⤳ Who Carries the Wood

In her day-to-day existence, a modern woman no longer experiences as strongly the feeling that a man is taking care of her. Sure, he is still going out and working hard for her, but she also is going out and working hard. Romance is anything that helps her to feel that she is not alone and that someone is there for her. Any little thing he can directly do for her says he cares and creates romance.

At one point Charley began asking Jeff, who helps with the yard once a month, to stack the wood for fires inside the house and set up a fire. When he would start these fires that Jeff built, he noticed that it didn't have the same effect on his wife as when he exerted himself and took the time to build the fire.

Intellectually, he could say, "I pay Jeff, so I should get the credit." But from Carol's emotional perspective, it didn't matter if Charley paid Jeff to do it. For romance to be created, sometimes a woman needs to directly experience her partner toiling for her.

This is a very important aspect of romantic rituals. Women like to see their men toil or make sacrifices for them. On a deep emotional level, if her husband carries in the heavy logs and takes the time to build a fire, she feels that he is exerting himself for her well-being, and she feels loved.

It is very different from exerting himself

for others who pay him and then bringing home the money. On an emotional level, when he is earning money, he is directing his attention and energy toward the people he works for and with and not toward her. For romance, a woman needs to feel a man's energy being spent and exerted directly for her.

❧

For romance, a woman needs to feel a man's energy being spent and exerted directly for her.

❧

❧ Taking Out the Trash

A woman particularly appreciates it when a man is happily willing to do something he really doesn't want to do. A great example of this is taking out the trash. Larry never used to take out the trash. But with Rose's persis-

tence in asking him to empty it in a nondemanding manner and then appreciating him
when he complied, his attitude changed.

Now whenever she seems a little distant
or frustrated, he starts looking to see if the
trash needs to be emptied. This response
happens because he repeatedly experienced how much she appreciates it when he
empties it. Not only does it help out, but it is
also a symbol of much more.

It says he is willing to come down off his
ladder of success and do what it takes to
make their life together work. It says he is
not above housework. It says she is not
alone, and he appreciates her efforts and is
willing to help lighten her heavy load. It
says he cares. When he gets home, he is now
happy to be the "maintenance man" for her.

∾ Helping with the Dishes

When Bonnie and I first got married, I told
her that I would be very involved in raising

our children and doing some housework, but I didn't like doing dishes.

I said, "I don't like doing dishes, and I don't want someone trying to make me feel guilty when I don't do them. If you don't like doing dishes, we can hire someone to do them."

She said it was fine and that she was happy doing them. When she was pregnant with our daughter Lauren, I could see that she was getting really exhausted doing dishes at night. I told her that for the rest of the pregnancy, I would do dishes, but that afterward we would go back to the old system.

Every night when I did the dishes, she was so appreciative. She treated me as if I was such a wonderful guy for doing them. A few months after Lauren was born, I very happily handed the job back to her. Again she was very appreciative that I had done it for so many months and didn't at all mind taking it back.

Well, after a few weeks, I began to miss how wonderful it felt when she appreciated me for doing the dishes. I would wait for her to look tired and then I would come in and offer to help. Each time, she was so happy and relieved.

Now, many years later I do dishes much of the time. Doing dishes is a way I can instantly get her love. She never takes it for granted and always appreciates me.

One day, someone asked my kids who does the dishes the most. They unanimously said me. Bonnie said she did, and the kids argued. I explained to the kids that she did the dishes more but that there was a good reason they thought I did.

In a playful manner, I said, "I only do dishes when someone can see me." Like any other romantic ritual, doing dishes is a little way I can help her and she can appreciate me. I do the dishes as a way to fill up with Bonnie's appreciation as well as to help.

∽ Doing Dishes Is Great Foreplay

Sometimes when my wife is really tired and goes to bed without cleaning the kitchen, I will stay and do the dishes. It rarely takes more than twenty or thirty minutes. When she gets up the next morning and finds a clean kitchen, she feels an incredible mixture of joy and relief. In an instant, her love for me dramatically goes up.

On many occasions, she has come back upstairs to awaken me in a most delightful manner. She whispers in my ear, "Was that you who cleaned the kitchen?" I smile and say, "Um-hum." She smiles back and this provides me with a most enjoyable and pleasurable morning delight.

This does not mean that every time I do the dishes, she is supposed to have sex with me. That would not be romance. That would be a business deal.

Doing the dishes commonly turns into sex because it makes her feel loved. Naturally, she begins to feel turned on. Knowing how much she appreciates my help makes doing the dishes a fulfilling activity for me as well.

∾ Going to Cultural Events

Grant and Theresa go to cultural events as a romantic ritual. Both Grant and Theresa enjoy going to the movies, but sometimes Theresa also likes to go to the theater or a concert. It took years before Grant realized how important it was for her to attend something besides just movies. He thought that since he was having such a good time at the movies, she was too.

She enjoyed going to the movies, but she also wanted to do other things. Now their romantic ritual is for her to mention certain events, and then he takes charge and schedules a date and buys the tickets.

All she has to say is that there is a new play in town, and he will take the hint and plan a date. He might say, "That sounds like a good idea. Let's go next Thursday night." When he makes a date in this way, she feels loved, romanced, and taken care of.

∽ Giving Compliments

Another little ritual is to compliment a woman whenever she gets dressed up, wears something different, or in any way seems to have put some effort into how she looks. Women can become very frustrated when men don't notice.

While Lucille was taking more time to get ready to go out, her husband, Steve, would wait downstairs. Then she would walk down the stairs and, instead of rushing, she would stop in the middle of the stairs for Steve to look at her and appreciate her beauty.

He didn't understand this female ritual and instead of complimenting her, he would say, "Come on, we're late." This did not go over well.

Eventually, she decided to help him out. The next time, when Lucille paused on the stairs, she said, "How do I look?"

Still not realizing the importance of this question, Steve said, "You look fine. Come on, we're late."

Again this didn't go over well. As Steve finally started learning about how men and women are different, he eventually realized his mistake.

Now when she comes down the stairs, he takes the time to notice how beautiful she is. Here is a list of expressive phrases men can use to most effectively compliment a woman:

"You look so beautiful."

"You look really great tonight."

"I love how you look in that dress."

"You look really wonderful."

"Fabulous, fabulous."

"You look great."

"I love the way you look tonight."

"You look really good."

"Your earrings are really great."

"I really love your colors."

"You look so spectacular."

"You are amazingly beautiful."

"You are so stunning."

"You really look sexy tonight."

"I love your legs."

"You are so radiant."

"You look really very lovely tonight."

"You are so gorgeous."

"You look so exquisite."

With each of these compliments, don't hesitate to add lots of embellishments, like *"really* beautiful," *"very* beautiful," or "so beautiful."

೨ The Power of Touch

A man reaching out to touch or hold hands is a turn-on for women. While men generally hold hands in the courting stage, they stop after a while. This is a big loss. A woman loves to feel that a man wants to connect with her in this way. She doesn't feel loved if the only time he wants to touch her is when he wants sex.

೨

A woman doesn't feel loved if the only time a man wants to touch her is when he wants sex.

೨

If a man wants his partner to feel receptive to sex, he needs to touch her in an affectionate way many times each day when he is not wanting sex. He can hold hands, put his arm around her, stroke her shoulders and arms, all without implying that he is wanting sex. If the only time he touches her is when he wants sex, she begins to feel used or taken for granted.

∼

If the only time he touches her is when he wants sex, she begins to feel used or taken for granted.

∼

When he is holding her hand, he should remember to be attentive. Many times a man will forget he is holding her hand and she is left holding a limp, lifeless hand. When he needs to shift his attention, he should just release her hand. She doesn't want to hold hands *all* the time. It is just a way to connect for a few minutes.

When I started being more affectionate and touching Bonnie more of the time, it made a tremendous difference. I couldn't believe that one simple little shift could have such a big influence. I had heard that women need to be touched twenty times a day in a nonsexual way to build high self-esteem. When I heard this, I thought I would experiment. I started out with ten times a day, and it worked great. Immediately, she began to shine more. Now I am much more affectionate when I am around her.

In the beginning, I did it just because I knew she liked it. Each time I would touch her, I could clearly sense that she was drinking it up. She loved it. I thought, "What a great discovery." Then as time passed, I started to really enjoy it myself.

Not only is touching her a great way to connect and feel close at any time, but it also softens the rough edges at times and brings us back to feeling our love for each other.

∽ Lasting Love, Romance, and Sex

All these romantic rituals are simple but powerful. They assist us in reconnecting with those very special feelings of attraction and passion that we can only feel when we are emotionally connected. These rituals ensure that the man can always do something to win his partner's love, and the woman can get the special attention and support she needs to stay passionately attracted to her partner.

∽

These rituals ensure that the man can always do something to win his partner's love, and the woman can get the special attention and support she needs to stay passionately attracted to her partner.

∽

By keeping the romance alive and practicing advanced bedroom skills, you can and will continue to enjoy great sex. May you always grow in love and passion and enjoy God's special gift. You deserve it.

If you like what you just read and want to learn more . . .

Every day we receive hundreds of phone calls and letters from readers asking for information regarding seminars, books, tapes, and other services. You can now call our representatives, Personal Growth Productions, twenty-four hours a day, seven days a week, toll free, at 1-888-MARSVENUS (1-888-627-7836) for information on the following subjects:

SEMINARS

More than 500,000 individuals and couples around the world have already benefited from John Gray's relationship seminars. We invite and encourage you to share with John this safe, insightful, and healing experience.

Because of the popularity of his seminars, Dr. Gray has developed programs for presentation by individuals he has personally trained and appointed. These seminars are available for both the general public as well as private corporate functions. This broad range of seminar opportunities continues to provide cherished memories and unforgettable experiences for attendees.

Please call for current schedules or booking information.

MARS/VENUS WORKSHOPS

The Mars/Venus Institute was created to offer workshops that bring Dr. Gray's information to local communities around the world. These exciting seminars feature John's favorite video segments and exercises presented by trained facilitators that have completed an in-depth course of study. Participants take home positive, practical experience that allows them to use Dr. Gray's suggestions comfortably and naturally. If you are interested in improving communication and developing more satisfying relationships, just give us a call and ask about Mars/Venus workshops.

MARS/VENUS COUNSELING CENTERS

No matter how helpful the insights in a book, tape, or seminar may be, they cannot replace the value of counseling and therapy. In response to the thousands of requests we have received for licensed professionals that use the Mars/Venus principles in their practice, Dr. Gray has established Mars/Venus Counseling Centers and Counselor Training. Participants in this program have completed an in-depth study of John's work and have demonstrated a commitment to his valuable concepts. If you are interested in a referral to a counselor in your area or information about training as a Mars/Venus counselor or establishing a Mars/Venus counseling center, please give us a call.

THE INTERNET

Visit John Gray's website at http://www. marsvenus.com. Ask questions about *Men Are from Mars, Women Are from Venus*. Chat with other Martians and Venusians. Shop for books, audiotapes, and videos.

Videos, Audiotapes, and Books by John Gray

For further exploration of the wonderful world of Mars and Venus, see the descriptions that follow and call us to place an order or for additional information.

If you like what you just read . . .

Personal Growth Productions
P.O. Box 51281
Phoenix, AZ 85076-51281
1-888-MARSVENUS (1-888-627-7836)
or 1-800-821-3033

VIDEOS

Men Are from Mars, Women Are from Venus
Twelve VHS cassettes

This is a complete collection of John Gray's work on video. In this series, Dr. Gray shares the insights and tools necessary for understanding, accepting, and loving our differences. In a positive and uplifting way, couples and singles learn to improve communication and enjoy healthy, happy relationships without sacrifice. Average running time is fifty minutes.

If you like what you just read . . .

Mars and Venus on a Date
Two VHS cassettes

After years of focusing on couples, Dr. Gray finally answers the thousands of singles and dating partners who asked him, "What about me?" John examines his five stages of dating: attraction, uncertainty, exclusivity, intimacy, and engagement. Find out why women need reassurance and men need encouragement. Increase your understanding of male/female differences and women's most asked question, "Why don't men commit?"

Men Are from Mars, Women Are from Venus—Children Are from Heaven
Two VHS cassettes

Dr. Gray lends his insights to parents trying to understand their little Martians and Venusians. In these cassettes you'll learn the five most important messages to give your children: It's Okay to Be Different; It's Okay to

Make Mistakes; It's Okay to Have Feelings; It's Okay to Ask for What You Want; It's Okay to Say No, But Mom and Dad Are the Boss.

AUDIOTAPES

Secrets of Successful Relationships
Twelve 45-minute audiocassettes

This audio series was taped live at Dr. Gray's two-and-a-half-day seminars and features three themes: The Secrets of Communication; Getting the Love You Deserve; and The Secrets of Intimacy and Passion.

Healing the Heart
Twelve 45-minute audiocassettes

The text and exercises contained in these tapes were originally taught as a week-long seminar designed to help individuals understand how and why the past affects the way they respond in relationships today. You will have the opportunity to create your own counseling sessions with the nation's leading expert on relationships and communication, and enjoy the benefits of healing your significant issues any time you choose.

⌒ **Available from the HarperCollins/ John Gray Collection at a retailer near you:**

**WHAT YOU FEEL, YOU CAN HEAL
A Guide for Enriching Relationships**

Two audiocassettes 0-69451-589-2 $17.00

**MEN, WOMEN AND RELATIONSHIPS
Making Peace with the Opposite Sex**

Paperback 0-06-101070-7 $6.99
One audiocassette 0-69451-534-5 $12.00

If you like what you just read . . .

MARS AND VENUS IN THE BEDROOM
A Guide to Lasting Romance and Passion

Hardcover 0-06-017212-6 $22.00
Two audiocassettes 0-69451-487-X $16.00

MARTE Y VENUS EN EL DORMITORIO
(SPANISH EDITION)

Trade paperback 0-06-095180-X $10.00
Two audiocassettes 0-69451-676-7 $18.00

THE MARS AND VENUS AUDIO COLLECTION

Contains one of each cassette: *Men Are from Mars, Women Are from Venus; What Your Mother Couldn't Tell You & Your Father Didn't Know;* and *Mars and Venus in the Bedroom*
Three audiocassettes 0-69451-589-2 $39.00

MARS AND VENUS TOGETHER FOREVER
Relationship Skills for Lasting Love

Trade paperback 0-06-092661-9 $13.00

If you like what you just read . . .

**MARTE Y VENUS JUNTOS PARA SIEMPRE
(SPANISH EDITION)**
Trade paperback 0-06-095236-9 $10.00

**MARS AND VENUS IN LOVE
Inspiring and Heartfelt Stories of
Relationships That Work**

Hardcover 0-06-017471-4 $18.00
One audiocassette 0-069451-713-5 $12.00